TO ERR IS HUMAN

Building a Safer Health System

Linda T. Kohn, Janet M. Corrigan, and
Molla S. Donaldson, *Editors*

Committee on Quality of Health Care in America

INSTITUTE OF MEDICINE

NATIONAL ACADEMY PRESS
Washington, D.C.

NATIONAL ACADEMY PRESS • 2101 Constitution Avenue, N.W. • Washington, DC 20418

NOTICE: The project that is the subject of this report was approved by the Governing Board of the National Research Council, whose members are drawn from the councils of the National Academy of Sciences, the National Academy of Engineering, and the Institute of Medicine. The members of the committee responsible for the report were chosen for their special competences and with regard for appropriate balance.

Support for this project was provided by The National Research Council and The Commonwealth Fund. The views presented in this report are those of the Institute of Medicine Committee on the Quality of Health Care in America and are not necessarily those of the funding agencies.

Library of Congress Cataloging-in-Publication Data

To err is human : building a safer health system / Linda T. Kohn, Janet M. Corrigan, and Molla S. Donaldson, editors.
   p. cm
   Includes bibliographical references and index.
   ISBN 0-309-06837-1
   1. Medical errors—Prevention. I. Kohn, Linda T. II. Corrigan, Janet. III.
Donaldson, Molla S.
R729.8.T6 2000
362.1—dc21   99-088993

Additional copies of this report are available for sale from the National Academy Press, 2101 Constitution Avenue, N.W., Box 285, Washington, DC 20055; call (800) 624-6242 or (202) 334-3313 in the Washington metropolitan area, or visit the NAP on-line bookstore at **www.nap.edu**.

The full text of this report is available on line at **www.nap.edu/readingroom.**

For more information about the Institute of Medicine, visit the IOM home page at **www.iom.edu.**

The serpent has been a symbol of long life, healing, and knowledge among almost all cultures and religions since the beginning of recorded history. The serpent adopted as a logotype by the Institute of Medicine is a relief carving from ancient Greece, now held by the Staatliche Museen in Berlin.

THE NATIONAL ACADEMIES

National Academy of Sciences
National Academy of Engineering
Institute of Medicine
National Research Council

The **National Academy of Sciences** is a private, nonprofit, self-perpetuating society of distinguished scholars engaged in scientific and engineering research, dedicated to the furtherance of science and technology and to their use for the general welfare. Upon the authority of the charter granted to it by the Congress in 1863, the Academy has a mandate that requires it to advise the federal government on scientific and technical matters. Dr. Bruce M. Alberts is president of the National Academy of Sciences.

The **National Academy of Engineering** was established in 1964, under the charter of the National Academy of Sciences, as a parallel organization of outstanding engineers. It is autonomous in its administration and in the selection of its members, sharing with the National Academy of Sciences the responsibility for advising the federal government. The National Academy of Engineering also sponsors engineering programs aimed at meeting national needs, encourages education and research, and recognizes the superior achievements of engineers. Dr. William A. Wulf is president of the National Academy of Engineering.

The **Institute of Medicine** was established in 1970 by the National Academy of Sciences to secure the services of eminent members of appropriate professions in the examination of policy matters pertaining to the health of the public. The Institute acts under the responsibility given to the National Academy of Sciences by its congressional charter to be an adviser to the federal government and, upon its own initiative, to identify issues of medical care, research, and education. Dr. Kenneth I. Shine is president of the Institute of Medicine.

The **National Research Council** was organized by the National Academy of Sciences in 1916 to associate the broad community of science and technology with the Academy's purposes of furthering knowledge and advising the federal government. Functioning in accordance with general policies determined by the Academy, the Council has become the principal operating agency of both the National Academy of Sciences and the National Academy of Engineering in providing services to the government, the public, and the scientific and engineering communities. The Council is administered jointly by both Academies and the Institute of Medicine. Dr. Bruce M. Alberts and Dr. William A. Wulf are chairman and vice chairman, respectively, of the National Research Council.

Study Staff

JANET M. CORRIGAN, Director, Division of Health Care Services,
    Director, Quality of Health Care in America Project
MOLLA S. DONALDSON, Project Co-Director
LINDA T. KOHN, Project Co-Director
TRACY McKAY, Research Assistant
KELLY C. PIKE, Senior Project Assistant

Auxiliary Staff

MIKE EDINGTON, Managing Editor
KAY C. HARRIS, Financial Advisor
SUZANNE MILLER, Senior Project Assistant

Copy Editor

FLORENCE POILLON

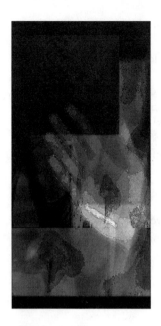

Reviewers

This report has been reviewed in draft form by individuals chosen for their diverse perspectives and technical expertise, in accordance with procedures approved by the National Research Council's Report Review Committee. The purpose of this independent review is to provide candid and critical comments that will assist the Institute of Medicine in making the published report as sound as possible and to ensure that the report meets institutional standards for objectivity, evidence, and responsiveness to the study charge. The review comments and the draft manuscript remain confidential to protect the integrity of the deliberative process. The committee wishes to thank the following individuals for their participation in the review of this report:

GERALDINE BEDNASH, Executive Director, American Association of
    Colleges of Nursing, Washington, DC
PETER BOUXSEIN, Visiting Scholar, Institute of Medicine, Washington,
    DC
JOHN COLMERS, Executive Director, Maryland Health Care Cost and
    Access Commission, Baltimore
JEFFREY COOPER, Director, Partners Biomedical Engineering Group,
    Massachusetts General Hospital, Boston
ROBERT HELMREICH, Professor, University of Texas at Austin

LOIS KERCHER, Vice President for Nursing, Sentara-Virginia Beach
    General Hospital, Virginia Beach, VA
GORDON MOORE, Associate Chief Medical Officer, Strong Health,
Rochester, NY
ALAN NELSON, Associate Executive Vice President, American College of
    Physicians/American Society of Internal Medicine, Washington, DC
LEE NEWCOMER, Chief Medical Officer, United HealthCare Corporation,
    Minnetonka, MN
MARY JANE OSBORN, University of Connecticut Health Center
ELLISON PIERCE, Executive Director, Anesthesia Patient Safety
    Foundation, Boston

Although the individuals acknowledged have provided valuable comments and suggestions, responsibility for the final contents of the report rests solely with the authoring committee and the Institute of Medicine.

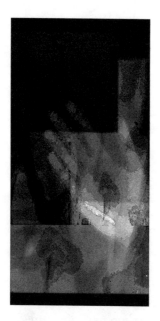

Preface

To *Err Is Human: Building a Safer Health System*. The title of this report encapsulates its purpose. Human beings, in all lines of work, make errors. Errors can be prevented by designing systems that make it hard for people to do the wrong thing and easy for people to do the right thing. Cars are designed so that drivers cannot start them while in reverse because that prevents accidents. Work schedules for pilots are designed so they don't fly too many consecutive hours without rest because alertness and performance are compromised.

In health care, building a safer system means designing processes of care to ensure that patients are safe from accidental injury. When agreement has been reached to pursue a course of medical treatment, patients should have the assurance that it will proceed correctly and safely so they have the best chance possible of achieving the desired outcome.

This report describes a serious concern in health care that, if discussed at all, is discussed only behind closed doors. As health care and the system that delivers it become more complex, the opportunities for errors abound. Correcting this will require a concerted effort by the professions, health care organizations, purchasers, consumers, regulators and policy-makers. Traditional clinical boundaries and a culture of blame must be broken down. But most importantly, we must systematically design safety into processes of care.

This report is part of larger project examining the quality of health care in America and how to achieve a threshold change in quality. The committee has focused its initial attention on quality concerns that fall into the category of medical errors. There are several reasons for this. First, errors are responsible for an immense burden of patient injury, suffering and death. Second, errors in the provision of health services, whether they result in injury or expose the patient to the risk of injury, are events that everyone agrees just shouldn't happen. Third, errors are readily understandable to the American public. Fourth, there is a sizable body of knowledge and very successful experiences in other industries to draw upon in tackling the safety problems of the health care industry. Fifth, the health care delivery system is rapidly evolving and undergoing substantial redesign, which may introduce improvements, but also new hazards. Over the next year, the committee will be examining other quality issues, such as problems of overuse and underuse.

The Quality of Health Care in America project is largely supported with income from an endowment established within the IOM by the Howard Hughes Medical Institute and income from an endowment established for the National Research Council by the Kellogg Foundation. The Commonwealth Fund provided generous support for a workshop to convene medical, nursing and pharmacy professionals for input into this specific report. The National Academy for State Health Policy assisted by convening a focus group of state legislative and regulatory leaders to discuss patient safety.

Thirty-eight people were involved in producing this report. The Subcommittee on Creating an External Environment for Quality, under the direction of J. Cris Bisgard and Molly Joel Coye, dealt with a series of complex and sensitive issues, always maintaining a spirit of compromise and respect. Additionally the Subcommittee on Designing the Health System of the 21st Century, under the direction of Donald Berwick, had to balance the challenges faced by health care organizations with the need to continually push out boundaries and not accept limitations. Lastly, under the direction of Janet Corrigan, excellent staff support has been provided by Linda Kohn, Molla Donaldson, Tracy McKay, and Kelly Pike.

At some point in our lives, each of us will probably be a patient in the health care system. It is hoped that this report can serve as a call to action that will illuminate a problem to which we are all vulnerable.

William C. Richardson, Ph.D.
Chair
November 1999

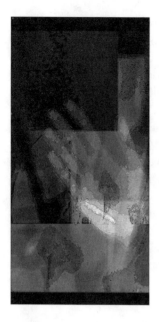

Foreword

This report is the first in a series of reports to be produced by the Quality of Health Care in America project. The Quality of Health Care in America project was initiated by the Institute of Medicine in June 1998 with the charge of developing a strategy that will result in a *threshold improvement* in quality over the next ten years.

Under the direction of Chairman William C. Richardson, the Quality of Health Care in America Committee is directed to:

- review and synthesize findings in the literature pertaining to the quality of care provided in the health care system;
- develop a communications strategy for raising the awareness of the general public and key stakeholders of quality of care concerns and opportunities for improvement;
- articulate a policy framework that will provide positive incentives to improve quality and foster accountability;
- identify characteristics and factors that enable or encourage providers, health care organizations, health plans and communities to continuously improve the quality of care; and
- develop a research agenda in areas of continued uncertainty.

This first report on patient safety addresses a serious issue affecting the quality of health care. Future reports in this series will address other quality-related issues and cover areas such as re-designing the health care delivery system for the 21st Century, aligning financial incentives to reward quality care and the critical role of information technology as a tool for measuring and understanding quality. Additional reports will be produced throughout the coming year.

The Quality of Health Care in America project continues IOM's long-standing focus on quality of care issues. The IOM National Roundtable on Health Care Quality described how variable the quality of health care is in this country and highlighted the urgent need for improving it. A recent report issued by the IOM National Cancer Policy Board concluded that there is a wide gulf between ideal cancer care and the reality that many Americans experience with cancer care.

The IOM will continue to call for a comprehensive and strong response to this most urgent issue facing the American people. This current report on patient safety further reinforces our conviction that we cannot wait any longer.

Kenneth I. Shine, M.D.
President, Institute of Medicine
November 1999

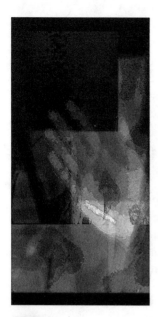

Acknowledgments

The Committee on the Quality of Health Care in America first and foremost acknowledges the tremendous contribution by the members of two subcommittees. Both subcommittees spent many hours working through a set of exceedingly complex issues, ranging from topics related to expectations from the health care delivery system to the details of how reporting systems work. Although individual subcommittee members raised different perspectives on a variety of issues, there was no disagreement on the ultimate goal of making care safer for patients. Without the efforts of the two subcommittees, this report would not have happened. We take this opportunity to thank each and every subcommittee member for their contribution.

SUBCOMMITTEE ON CREATING AN ENVIRONMENT FOR QUALITY IN HEALTH CARE

J. Cris Bisgard (*Cochair*), Delta Air Lines, Inc.; Molly Joel Coye, (*Cochair*), The Lewin Group; Phyllis C. Borzi, The George Washington University; Charles R. Buck, Jr., General Electric Company; Jon Christianson, University of Minnesota; Charles Cutler, formerly of The Prudential HealthCare; Mary Jane England, Washington Business Group on Health; George J. Isham, HealthPartners; Brent James, Intermountain Health Care; Roz D.

Lasker, New York Academy of Medicine; Lucian Leape, Harvard School of Public Health; Patricia A. Riley, National Academy of State Health Policy; Gerald M. Shea, American Federation of Labor and Congress of Industrial Organizations; Gail L. Warden, Henry Ford Health System; A. Eugene Washington, University of California, San Francisco School of Medicine; and Andrew Webber, Consumer Coalition for Health Care Quality.

SUBCOMMITTEE ON BUILDING THE 21ST CENTURY HEALTH CARE SYSTEM

Don M. Berwick (*Chair*), Institute for Healthcare Improvement; Christine K. Cassel, Mount Sinai School of Medicine; Rodney Dueck, HealthSystem Minnesota; Jerome H. Grossman, Lion Gate Management Corporation; John E. Kelsch, Consultant in Total Quality; Risa Lavizzo-Mourey, University of Pennsylvania; Arthur Levin, Center for Medical Consumers; Eugene C. Nelson, Hitchcock Medical Center; Thomas Nolan, Associates in Proc-ess Improvement; Gail J. Povar, Cameron Medical Group; James L. Reinertsen, CareGroup; Joseph E. Scherger, University of California, Irvine; Stephen M. Shortell, University of California, Berkeley; Mary Wakefield, George Mason University; and Kevin Weiss, Rush Primary Care Institute.

A number of people willingly and generously gave their time and expertise as the committee and both subcommittees conducted their deliberations. Their contributions are acknowledged here.

Participants in the Roundtable on the Role of the Health Professions in Improving Patient Safety provided many useful insights reflected in the final report. They included: J. Cris Bisgard, Delta Air Lines, Inc.; Terry P. Clemmer, Intermountain Health Care; Leo J. Dunn, Virginia Commonwealth University; James Espinosa, Overlook Hospital; Paul Friedmann, Bay State Hospital; David M. Gaba, V.A. Palo Alto HCS; Larry A. Green, American Academy of Family Physicians; Paul F. Griner, Association of American Medical Colleges; Charles Douglas Hepler, University of Florida; Carolyn Hutcherson, Health Policy Consultant; Lucian L. Leape, Harvard School of Public Health; William C. Nugent, Dartmouth Hitchcock Medical Center; Ellison C. Pierce Jr., Anesthesia Patient Safety Foundation; Bernard Rosof, Huntington Hospital; Carol Taylor, Georgetown University; Mary Wakefield, George Mason University; and Richard Womer, Children's Hospital of Philadelphia.

We are also grateful to the state representatives who participated in the focus group on patient safety convened by the National Academy for State Health Policy, including: Anne Barry, Minnesota Department of Finance; Jane Beyer, Washington State House of Representatives; Maureen Booth, National Academy of State Health Policy Fellow; Eileen Cody, Washington State House of Representatives; John Colmers, Maryland Health Care Access and Cost Commission; Patrick Finnerty, Virginia Joint Commission on Health Care; John Frazer, Delaware Office of the Controller General; Lori Gerhard, Commonwealth of Pennsylvania, Department of Health; Jeffrey Gregg, State of Florida, Agency for Health Care Administration; Frederick Heigel, New York Bureau of Hospital and Primary Care Services; John LaCour, Louisiana Department of Health and Hospitals; Maureen Maigret, Rhode Island Lieutenant Governor's Office; Angela Monson, Oklahoma State Senate; Catherine Morris, New Jersey State Department of Health; Danielle Noe, Kansas Office of the Governor; Susan Reinhard, New Jersey Department of Health and Senior Services; Trish Riley, National Academy for State Health Policy; Dan Rubin, Washington State Department of Health; Brent Ewig, ASTHO; Kathy Weaver, Indiana State Department of Health; and Robert Zimmerman, Pennsylvania Department of Health.

A number of people at the state health departments generously provided information about the adverse event reporting program in their state. The committee thanks the following people for their time and help: Karen Logan, California; Jackie Starr-Bocian, Colorado; Julie Moore, Connecticut; Anna Polk, Florida; Mary Kabril, Kansas; Lee Kelly, Massachusetts; Vanessa Phipps, Mississippi; Nancy Garvey, New Jersey; Ellen Flink, New York; Kathryn Kimmet, Ohio; Larry Stoller, Jim Steel and Elaine Gibble, Pennsylvania; Laurie Round, Rhode Island; and Connie Richards, South Dakota. In addition, Renee Mallett at the Ohio Hospital Association also offered assistance.

From the Food and Drug Administration, the Committee especially recognizes the contributions of Janet Woodcock, Director, Center for Drug Evaluation and Research; Ralph Lillie, Director, Office of Post-Marketing Drug Risk Assessment; Susan Gardner, Deputy Director, Center for Devices and Radiological Health; Jerry Phillips, Associate Director, Medication Error Program and Peter Carstenson, Senior Systems Engineer, Division of Device User Programs and System Analysis.

Assistance from the Agency for Healthcare Research and Quality came from John M. Eisenberg, Administrator; Gregg Meyer, Director of the Center for Quality Measurement and Improvement; Nancy Foster, Coordinator for Quality Activities and Marge Keyes, Project Officer. At the Health Care Financing Administration, Jeff Kang, Director, Clinical Standards and Quality and Tim Cuerdon, Office of Clinical Standards and Quality were especially helpful. At the Veterans Health Administration, Kenneth Kizer, former Undersecretary for Health and Ronald Goldman, Office of Performance and Quality shared their views on how to create a culture of safety inside large health care organizations.

Other individuals provided data, information and background that significantly contributed to the committee's understanding of patient safety. The committee would like to particularly acknowledge the contributions of Charles Billings, now at Ohio State University and designer of the Aviation Safety Reporting System; Linda Blank at the American Board of Internal Medicine; Michael Cohen at the Institute for Safe Medication Practices; Linda Connell at the Aviation Safety Reporting System at NASA/Ames Research Center; Diane Cousins and Fay Menacker at U.S. Pharmacopeia, Martin Hatlie and Eleanor Vogt at the National Patient Safety Foundation; Henry Manasse and Colleen O'Malley at the American Society of Health-System Pharmacists; Cynthia Null at the Human Factors Research and Technology Division at NASA/Ames Research Center; Eric Thomas, at the University of Texas at Houston; Margaret VanAmringe at the Joint Commission on Accreditation of Health Care Organizations; and Karen Williams at the National Pharmaceuticals Council.

A special thanks is offered to Randall R. Bovbjerg and David W. Shapiro for preparing a paper on the legal discovery of data reported to adverse event reporting systems. Their paper significantly contributed to Chapter 6 of this report, although the conclusions and findings are the full responsibility of the committee (readers should not interpret their input as legal advice nor representing the views of their employing organizations).

A special thanks is also provided to colleagues at the IOM. Claudia Carl and Mike Edington provided assistance during the report review and preparation stages. Ellen Agard and Mel Worth significantly contributed to the case study that is used in the report. Wilhelmine Miller expertly arranged the workshop with physicians, nurses and pharmacists and ensured a successful meeting. Suzanne Miller provided important assistance to the literature review. Tracy McKay provided help throughout the project, from coordinating literature searches to overseeing the editing of the report. A special thanks is offered to Kelly Pike. Her outstanding support and attention to detail was critical to the success of this report. Her assistance was always offered with enthusiasm and good cheer.

Finally, the committee acknowledges the generous support from the National Research Council and the Institute of Medicine to conduct this work. Additionally, the committee thanks Brian Biles for his interest in this work and gratefully acknowledges the contribution of The Commonwealth Fund, a New York City-based private independent foundation. The views presented here are those of the authors and not necessarily those of The Commonwealth Fund, its directors, officers or staff.

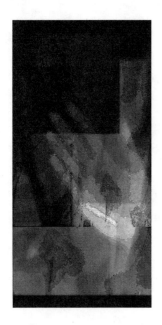

Contents

Key Safety Design Concepts, 162
Principles for the Design of Safety Systems in
    Health Care Organizations, 165
Medication Safety, 182
Summary, 197

APPENDIXES

TO ERR IS HUMAN

Building a Safer Health System

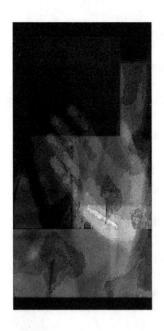

Executive
Summary

The knowledgeable health reporter for the *Boston Globe*, Betsy Lehman, died from an overdose during chemotherapy. Willie King had the wrong leg amputated. Ben Kolb was eight years old when he died during "minor" surgery due to a drug mix-up.[1]

These horrific cases that make the headlines are just the tip of the iceberg. Two large studies, one conducted in Colorado and Utah and the other in New York, found that adverse events occurred in 2.9 and 3.7 percent of hospitalizations, respectively.[2] In Colorado and Utah hospitals, 6.6 percent of adverse events led to death, as compared with 13.6 percent in New York hospitals. In both of these studies, over half of these adverse events resulted from medical errors and could have been prevented.

When extrapolated to the over 33.6 million admissions to U.S. hospitals in 1997, the results of the study in Colorado and Utah imply that at least 44,000 Americans die each year as a result of medical errors.[3] The results of the New York Study suggest the number may be as high as 98,000.[4] Even when using the lower estimate, deaths due to medical errors exceed the number attributable to the 8th-leading cause of death.[5] More people die in a given year as a result of medical errors than from motor vehicle accidents (43,458), breast cancer (42,297), or AIDS (16,516).[6]

Total national costs (lost income, lost household production, disability and health care costs) of preventable adverse events (medical errors resulting in injury) are estimated to be between $17 billion and $29 billion, of which health care costs represent over one-half.[7]

In terms of lives lost, patient safety is as important an issue as worker safety. Every year, over 6,000 Americans die from workplace injuries.[8] Medication errors alone, occurring either in or out of the hospital, are estimated to account for over 7,000 deaths annually.[9]

Medication-related errors occur frequently in hospitals and although not all result in actual harm, those that do, are costly. One recent study conducted at two prestigious teaching hospitals, found that about two out of every 100 admissions experienced a preventable adverse drug event, resulting in average increased hospital costs of $4,700 per admission or about $2.8 million annually for a 700-bed teaching hospital.[10] If these findings are generalizable, the increased hospital costs alone of preventable adverse drug events affecting inpatients are about $2 billion for the nation as a whole.

These figures offer only a very modest estimate of the magnitude of the problem since hospital patients represent only a small proportion of the total population at risk, and direct hospital costs are only a fraction of total costs. More care and increasingly complex care is provided in ambulatory settings. Outpatient surgical centers, physician offices and clinics serve thousands of patients daily. Home care requires patients and their families to use complicated equipment and perform follow-up care. Retail pharmacies play a major role in filling prescriptions for patients and educating them about their use. Other institutional settings, such as nursing homes, provide a broad array of services to vulnerable populations. Although many of the available studies have focused on the hospital setting, medical errors present a problem in any setting, not just hospitals.

Errors are also costly in terms of opportunity costs. Dollars spent on having to repeat diagnostic tests or counteract adverse drug events are dollars unavailable for other purposes. Purchasers and patients pay for errors when insurance costs and copayments are inflated by services that would not have been necessary had proper care been provided. It is impossible for the nation to achieve the greatest value possible from the billions of dollars spent on medical care if the care contains errors.

But not all the costs can be directly measured. Errors are also costly in terms of loss of trust in the system by patients and diminished satisfaction by both patients and health professionals. Patients who experience a longer hospital stay or disability as a result of errors pay with physical and psychological discomfort. Health care professionals pay with loss of morale and frustration at not being able to provide the best care possible. Employers and society, in general, pay in terms of lost worker productivity, reduced school attendance by children, and lower levels of population health status. Yet silence surrounds this issue. For the most part, consumers believe they are protected. Media coverage has been limited to reporting of anecdotal cases. Licensure and accreditation confer, in the eyes of the public, a "Good Housekeeping Seal of Approval." Yet, licensing and accreditation processes have focused only limited attention on the issue, and even these minimal efforts have confronted some resistance from health care organizations and providers. Providers also perceive the medical liability system as a serious impediment to systematic efforts to uncover and learn from errors.[11]

The decentralized and fragmented nature of the health care delivery system (some would say "nonsystem") also contributes to unsafe conditions for patients, and serves as an impediment to efforts to improve safety. Even within hospitals and large medical groups, there are rigidly-defined areas of specialization and influence. For example, when patients see multiple providers in different settings, none of whom have access to complete information, it is easier for something to go wrong than when care is better coordinated. At the same time, the provision of care to patients by a collection of loosely affiliated organizations and providers makes it difficult to implement improved clinical information systems capable of providing timely access to complete patient information. Unsafe care is one of the prices we pay for not having organized systems of care with clear lines of accountability.

Lastly, the context in which health care is purchased further exacerbates these problems. Group purchasers have made few demands for improvements in safety.[12] Most third party payment systems provide little incentive for a health care organization to improve safety, nor do they recognize and reward safety or quality.

The goal of this report is to break this cycle of inaction. The status quo is not acceptable and cannot be tolerated any longer. Despite the cost pressures, liability constraints, resistance to change and other seemingly insurmountable barriers, it is simply not acceptable for patients to be harmed by the same health care system that is supposed to offer healing and comfort. "First do no harm" is an often quoted term from Hippocrates.[13] Everyone working in health care is familiar with the term. At a very minimum, the health system needs to offer that assurance and security to the public.

A comprehensive approach to improving patient safety is needed. This approach cannot focus on a single solution since there is no "magic bullet" that will solve this problem, and indeed, no single recommendation in this report should be considered as *the* answer. Rather, large, complex problems require thoughtful, multifaceted responses. The combined goal of the recommendations is for the external environment to create sufficient pressure to make errors costly to health care organizations and providers, so they are compelled to take action to improve safety. At the same time, there is a need to enhance knowledge and tools to improve safety and break down legal and cultural barriers that impede safety improvement. Given current knowledge about the magnitude of the problem, the committee believes it would be irresponsible to expect anything less than a 50 percent reduction in errors over five years.

In this report, safety is defined as freedom from accidental injury. This definition recognizes that this is the primary safety goal from the patient's perspective. Error is defined as the failure of a planned action to be completed as intended or the use of a wrong plan to achieve an aim. According to noted expert James Reason, errors depend on two kinds of failures: either the correct action does not proceed as intended (an error of execution) or the original intended action is not correct (an error of planning).[14] Errors can happen in all stages in the process of care, from diagnosis, to treatment, to preventive care.

Not all errors result in harm. Errors that do result in injury are sometimes called preventable adverse events. An adverse event is an injury resulting from a medical intervention, or in other words, it is not due to the underlying condition of the patient. While all adverse events result from medical management, not all are preventable (i.e., not all are attributable to errors). For example, if a patient has surgery and dies from pneumonia he or she got postoperatively, it is an adverse event. If analysis of the case reveals that the patient got pneumonia because of poor hand washing or instrument cleaning techniques by staff, the adverse event was preventable (attributable to an error of execution). But the analysis may conclude that no error occurred and the patient would be presumed to have had a difficult surgery and recovery (not a preventable adverse event).

Much can be learned from the analysis of errors. All adverse events resulting in serious injury or death should be evaluated to assess whether improvements in the delivery system can be made to reduce the likelihood of similar events occurring in the future. Errors that do not result in harm also represent an important opportunity to identify system improvements having the potential to prevent adverse events. Preventing errors means designing the health care system at all levels to make it safer. Building safety into processes of care is a more effective way to reduce errors than blaming individuals (some experts, such as Deming, believe improving processes is the only way to improve quality[15]). The focus must shift from blaming individuals for past errors to a focus on preventing future errors by designing safety into the system. This does not mean that individuals can be careless. People must still be vigilant and held responsible for their actions. But when an error occurs, blaming an individual does little to make the system safer and prevent someone else from committing the same error.

Health care is a decade or more behind other high-risk industries in its attention to ensuring basic safety. Aviation has focused extensively on building safe systems and has been doing so since World War II. Between 1990 and 1994, the U.S. airline fatality rate was less than one-third the rate experienced in mid century.[16] In 1998, there were no deaths in the United States in commercial aviation. In health care, preventable injuries from care have been estimated to affect between three to four percent of hospital patients.[17] Although health care may never achieve aviation's impressive record, there is clearly room for improvement.

To err is human, but errors can be prevented. Safety is a critical first step in improving quality of care. The Harvard Medical Practice Study, a seminal research study on this issue, was published almost ten years ago; other studies have corroborated its findings. Yet few tangible actions to improve patient safety can be found. Must we wait another decade to be safe in our health system?

RECOMMENDATIONS

The IOM Quality of Health Care in America Committee was formed in June 1998 to develop a strategy that will result in a threshold improvement in quality over the next ten years. This report addresses issues related to patient safety, a subset of overall quality-related concerns, and lays out a national agenda for reducing errors in health care and improving patient safety. Although it is a national agenda, many activities are aimed at prompting responses at the state and local levels and within health care organizations and professional groups.

The committee believes that although there is still much to learn about the types of errors committed in health care and why they occur, enough is known today to recognize that a serious concern exists for patients. Whether a person is sick or just trying to stay healthy, they should not have to worry about being harmed by the health system itself. This report is a call to action to make health care safer for patients.

The committee believes that a major force for improving patient safety is the intrinsic motivation of health care providers, shaped by professional ethics, norms and expectations. But the interaction between factors in the external environment and factors inside health care organizations can also prompt the changes needed to improve patient safety. Factors in the external environment include availability of knowledge and tools to improve safety, strong and visible professional leadership, legislative and regulatory initiatives, and actions of purchasers and consumers to demand safety improvements. Factors inside health care organizations include strong leadership for safety, an organizational culture that encourages recognition and learning from errors, and an effective patient safety program.

In developing its recommendations, the committee seeks to strike a balance between regulatory and market-based initiatives, and between the roles of professionals and organizations. No single action represents a complete answer, nor can any single group or sector offer a complete fix to the problem. However, different groups can, and should, make significant contributions to the solution. The committee recognizes that a number of groups are already working on improving patient safety, such as the National Patient Safety Foundation and the Anesthesia Patient Safety Foundation.

The recommendations contained in this report lay out a four-tiered approach:

- establishing a national focus to create leadership, research, tools and protocols to enhance the knowledge base about safety;
- identifying and learning from errors through immediate and strong mandatory reporting efforts, as well as the encouragement of voluntary efforts, both with the aim of making sure the system continues to be made safer for patients;
- raising standards and expectations for improvements in safety through the actions of oversight organizations, group purchasers, and professional groups; and
- creating safety systems inside health care organizations through the implementation of safe practices at the delivery level. This level is the ultimate target of all the recommendations.

Leadership and Knowledge

Other industries that have been successful in improving safety, such as aviation and occupational health, have had the support of a designated agency that sets and communicates priorities, monitors progress in achieving goals, directs resources toward areas of need, and brings visibility to important issues. Although various agencies and organizations in health care may contribute to certain of these activities, there is no focal point for raising and sustaining attention to patient safety. Without it, health care is unlikely to match the safety improvements achieved in other industries.

The growing awareness of the frequency and significance of errors in health care creates an imperative to improve our understanding of the problem and devise workable solutions. For some types of errors, the knowledge of how to prevent them exists today. In these areas, the need is for widespread dissemination of this information. For other areas, however, additional work is needed to develop and apply the knowledge that will make care safer for patients. Resources invested in building the knowledge base and diffusing the expertise throughout the industry can pay large dividends to both patients and the health professionals caring for them and produce savings for the health system.

RECOMMENDATION 4.1 Congress should create a Center for Patient Safety within the Agency for Healthcare Research and Quality. This center should

- **set the national goals for patient safety, track progress in meeting these goals, and issue an annual report to the President and Congress on patient safety; and**
- **develop knowledge and understanding of errors in health care by developing a research agenda, funding Centers of Excellence, evaluating methods for identifying and preventing errors, and funding dissemination and communication activities to improve patient safety.**

To make significant improvements in patient safety, a highly visible center is needed, with secure and adequate funding. The Center should establish goals for safety; develop a research agenda; define prototype safety systems; develop and disseminate tools for identifying and analyzing errors and evaluate approaches taken; develop tools and methods for educating consumers about patient safety; issue an annual report on the state of patient safety, and recommend additional improvements as needed.

The committee recommends initial annual funding for the Center of $30 to $35 million. This initial funding would permit a center to conduct activities in goal setting, tracking, research and dissemination. Funding should grow over time to at least $100 million, or approximately 1% of the $8.8 billion in health care costs attributable to preventable adverse events.[18]

This initial level of funding is modest relative to the resources devoted to other public health issues. The Center for Patient Safety should be created within the Agency for Healthcare Research and Quality because the agency is already involved in a broad range of quality and safety issues, and has established the infrastructure and experience to fund research, educational and coordinating activities.

Identifying and Learning from Errors

Another critical component of a comprehensive strategy to improve patient safety is to create an environment that encourages organizations to identify errors, evaluate causes and take appropriate actions to improve performance in the future. External reporting systems represent one mechanism to enhance our understanding of errors and the underlying factors that contribute to them.

Reporting systems can be designed to meet two purposes. They can be designed as part of a public system for holding health care organizations accountable for performance. In this instance, reporting is often mandatory, usually focuses on specific cases that involve serious harm or death, may result in fines or penalties relative to the specific case, and information about the event may become known to the public. Such systems ensure a response to specific reports of serious injury, hold organizations and providers accountable for maintaining safety, respond to the public's right to know, and provide incentives to health care organizations to implement internal safety systems that reduce the likelihood of such events occurring. Currently, at least twenty states have mandatory adverse event reporting systems.

Voluntary, confidential reporting systems can also be part of an overall program for improving patient safety and can be designed to complement the mandatory reporting systems previously described. Voluntary reporting systems, which generally focus on a much broader set of errors and strive to detect system weaknesses before the occurrence of serious harm, can provide rich information to health care organizations in support of their quality improvement efforts.

For either purpose, the goal of reporting systems is to analyze the information they gather and identify ways to prevent future errors from occurring. The goal is not data collection. Collecting reports and not doing anything with the information serves no useful purpose. Adequate resources and other support must be provided for analysis and response to critical issues.

RECOMMENDATION 5.1 A nationwide mandatory reporting system should be established that provides for the collection of standardized information by state governments about adverse events that result in death or serious harm. Reporting should initially be required of hospitals and eventually be required of other institutional and ambulatory care delivery settings. Congress should

• designate the National Forum for Health Care Quality Measurement and Reporting as the entity responsible for promulgating and maintaining a core set of reporting standards to be used by states, including a nomenclature and taxonomy for reporting;
• require all health care organizations to report standardized information on a defined list of adverse events;
• provide funds and technical expertise for state governments to establish or adapt their current error reporting systems to collect the standardized information, analyze it and conduct follow-up action as needed with health care organizations. Should a state choose not to implement the mandatory reporting system, the Department of Health and Human Services should be designated as the responsible entity; and
• designate the Center for Patient Safety to:

(1) convene states to share information and expertise, and to evaluate alternative approaches taken for implementing reporting programs, identify best practices for implementation, and assess the impact of state programs; and
(2) receive and analyze aggregate reports from states to identify persistent safety issues that require more intensive analysis and/or a broader-based response (e.g., designing prototype systems or requesting a response by agencies, manufacturers or others).

RECOMMENDATION 5.2 The development of voluntary reporting efforts should be encouraged. The Center for Patient Safety should

• describe and disseminate information on external voluntary reporting programs to encourage greater participation in them and track the development of new reporting systems as they form;
• convene sponsors and users of external reporting systems to evaluate what works and what does not work well in the programs, and ways to make them more effective;
• periodically assess whether additional efforts are needed to address gaps in information to improve patient safety and to encourage

health care organizations to participate in voluntary reporting programs; and
  • fund and evaluate pilot projects for reporting systems, both within individual health care organizations and collaborative efforts among health care organizations.

The committee believes there is a role both for mandatory, public reporting systems and voluntary, confidential reporting systems. However, because of their distinct purposes, such systems should be operated and maintained separately. A nationwide mandatory reporting system should be established by building upon the current patchwork of state systems and by standardizing the types of adverse events and information to be reported. The newly established National Forum for Health Care Quality Measurement and Reporting, a public/private partnership, should be charged with the establishment of such standards. Voluntary reporting systems should also be promoted and the participation of health care organizations in them should be encouraged by accrediting bodies.

RECOMMENDATION 6.1 Congress should pass legislation to extend peer review protections to data related to patient safety and quality improvement that are collected and analyzed by health care organizations for internal use or shared with others solely for purposes of improving safety and quality.

The committee believes that information about the most serious adverse events which result in harm to patients and which are subsequently found to result from errors should not be protected from public disclosure. However, the committee also recognizes that for events not falling under this category, fears about the legal discoverability of information may undercut motivations to detect and analyze errors to improve safety. Unless such data are assured protection, information about errors will continue to be hidden and errors will be repeated. A more conducive environment is needed to encourage health care professionals and organizations to identify, analyze, and report errors without threat of litigation and without compromising patients' legal rights.

Setting Performance Standards and Expectations for Safety

Setting and enforcing explicit standards for safety through regulatory and related mechanisms, such as licensing, certification, and accreditation, can define minimum performance levels for health care organizations and professionals. Additionally, the process of developing and adopting standards helps to form expectations for safety among providers and consumers. However, standards and expectations are not only set through regulations. The actions of purchasers and consumers affect the behaviors of health care organizations, and the values and norms set by health professions influence standards of practice, training and education for providers. Standards for patient safety can be applied to health care professionals, the organizations in which they work, and the tools (drugs and devices) they use to care for patients.

> **RECOMMENDATION 7.1 Performance standards and expectations for health care organizations should focus greater attention on patient safety.**
>
> • **Regulators and accreditors should require health care organizations to implement meaningful patient safety programs with defined executive responsibility.**
> • **Public and private purchasers should provide incentives to health care organizations to demonstrate continuous improvement in patient safety.**

Health care organizations are currently subject to compliance with licensing and accreditation standards. Although both devote some attention to issues related to patient safety, there is opportunity to strengthen such efforts. Regulators and accreditors have a role in encouraging and supporting actions in health care organizations by holding them accountable for ensuring a safe environment for patients. After a reasonable period of time for health care organizations to develop patient safety programs, regulators and accreditors should require them as a minimum standard.

Purchaser and consumer demands also exert influence on health care organizations. Public and private purchasers should consider safety issues in their contracting decisions and reinforce the importance of patient safety by providing relevant information to their employees or beneficiaries. Purchasers should also communicate concerns about patient safety to accrediting bodies to support stronger oversight for patient safety.

> **RECOMMENDATION 7.2 Performance standards and expectations for health professionals should focus greater attention on patient safety.**

- Health professional licensing bodies should

(1) implement periodic re-examinations and re-licensing of doctors, nurses, and other key providers, based on both competence and knowledge of safety practices; and
(2) work with certifying and credentialing organizations to develop more effective methods to identify unsafe providers and take action.

- Professional societies should make a visible commitment to patient safety by establishing a permanent committee dedicated to safety improvement. This committee should

(1) develop a curriculum on patient safety and encourage its adoption into training and certification requirements;
(2) disseminate information on patient safety to members through special sessions at annual conferences, journal articles and editorials, newsletters, publications and websites on a regular basis;
(3) recognize patient safety considerations in practice guidelines and in standards related to the introduction and diffusion of new technologies, therapies and drugs;
(4) work with the Center for Patient Safety to develop community-based, collaborative initiatives for error reporting and analysis and implementation of patient safety improvements; and
(5) collaborate with other professional societies and disciplines in a national summit on the professional's role in patient safety.

Although unsafe practitioners are believed to be few in number, the rapid identification of such practitioners and corrective action are important to a comprehensive safety program. Responsibilities for documenting continuing skills are dispersed among licensing boards, specialty boards and professional groups, and health care organizations with little communication or coordination. In their ongoing assessments, existing licensing, certification and accreditation processes for health professionals should place greater attention on safety and performance skills.

Additionally, professional societies and groups should become active leaders in encouraging and demanding improvements in patient safety. Setting standards, convening and communicating with members about safety, incorporating attention to patient safety into training programs and collaborating across disciplines are all mechanisms that will contribute to creating a culture of safety.

> **RECOMMENDATION 7.3** The Food and Drug Administration (FDA) should increase attention to the safe use of drugs in both pre- and post-marketing processes through the following actions:
>
> • develop and enforce standards for the design of drug packaging and labeling that will maximize safety in use;
> • require pharmaceutical companies to test (using FDA-approved methods) proposed drug names to identify and remedy potential sound-alike and look-alike confusion with existing drug names; and
> • work with physicians, pharmacists, consumers, and others to establish appropriate responses to problems identified through post-marketing surveillance, especially for concerns that are perceived to require immediate response to protect the safety of patients.

The FDA's role is to regulate manufacturers for the safety and effectiveness of their drugs and devices. However, even approved products can present safety problems in practice. For example, different drugs with similar sounding names can create confusion for both patients and providers. Attention to the safety of products in actual use should be increased during approval processes and in post-marketing monitoring systems. The FDA should also work with drug manufacturers, distributors, pharmacy benefit managers, health plans and other organizations to assist clinicians in identifying and preventing problems in the use of drugs.

Implementing Safety Systems in Health Care Organizations

Experience in other high-risk industries has provided well-understood illustrations that can be used to improve health care safety. However, health care management and professionals have rarely provided specific, clear, high-level, organization-wide incentives to apply what has been learned in other industries about ways to prevent error and reduce harm within their own organizations. Chief Executive Officers and Boards of Trustees should be held accountable for making a serious, visible and on-going commitment to creating safe systems of care.

RECOMMENDATION 8.1 Health care organizations and the professionals affiliated with them should make continually improved patient safety a declared and serious aim by establishing patient safety programs with defined executive responsibility. Patient safety programs should

- provide strong, clear and visible attention to safety;
- implement non-punitive systems for reporting and analyzing errors within their organizations;
- incorporate well-understood safety principles, such as standardizing and simplifying equipment, supplies, and processes; and
- establish interdisciplinary team training programs for providers that incorporate proven methods of team training, such as simulation.

Health care organizations must develop a culture of safety such that an organization's care processes and workforce are focused on improving the reliability and safety of care for patients. Safety should be an explicit organizational goal that is demonstrated by the strong direction and involvement of governance, management and clinical leadership. In addition, a meaningful patient safety program should include defined program objectives, personnel, and budget and should be monitored by regular progress reports to governance.

RECOMMENDATION 8.2 Health care organizations should implement proven medication safety practices.

A number of practices have been shown to reduce errors in the medication process. Several professional and collaborative organizations interested in patient safety have developed and published recommendations for safe medication practices, especially for hospitals. Although some of these recommendations have been implemented, none have been universally adopted and some are not yet implemented in a majority of hospitals. Safe medication practices should be implemented in all hospitals and health care organizations in which they are appropriate.

SUMMARY

This report lays out a comprehensive strategy for addressing a serious problem in health care to which we are all vulnerable. By laying out a concise list of recommendations, the committee does not underestimate the many barriers that must be overcome to accomplish this agenda. Significant changes are required to improve awareness of the problem by the public and health professionals, to align payment systems and the liability system so they encourage safety improvements, to develop training and education programs that emphasize the importance of safety and for chief executive officers and trustees of health care organizations to create a culture of safety and demonstrate it in their daily decisions.

Although no single activity can offer the solution, the combination of activities proposed offers a roadmap toward a safer health system. The proposed program should be evaluated after five years to assess progress in making the health system safer. With adequate leadership, attention and resources, improvements can be made. It may be part of human nature to err, but it is also part of human nature to create solutions, find better alternatives and meet the challenges ahead.

REFERENCES

1. Cook, Richard; Woods, David; Miller, Charlotte, *A Tale of Two Stories: Contrasting Views of Patient Safety.* Chicago: National Patient Safety Foundation, 1998.

2. Brennan, Troyen A.; Leape, Lucian L.; Laird, Nan M., et al. Incidence of adverse events and negligence in hospitalized patients: Results of the Harvard Medical Practice Study I. *N Engl J Med.* 324:370–376, 1991. See also: Leape, Lucian L.; Brennan, Troyen A.; Laird, Nan M., et al. The Nature of Adverse Events in Hospitalized Patients: Results of the Harvard Medical Practice Study II. *N Engl J Med.* 324(6):377–384, 1991. See also: Thomas, Eric J.; Studdert, David M.; Burstin, Helen R., et al. Incidence and Types of Adverse Events and Negligent Care in Utah and Colorado. *Med Care* forthcoming Spring 2000.

3. American Hospital Association. Hospital Statistics. Chicago. 1999. See also: Thomas, Eric J.; Studdert, David M.; Burstin, Helen R., et al. Incidence and Types of Adverse Events and Negligent Care in Utah and Colorado. *Med Care* forthcoming Spring 2000. See also: Thomas, Eric J.; Studdert, David M.; Newhouse, Joseph P., et al. Costs of Medical Injuries in Utah and Colorado. *Inquiry.* 36:255–264, 1999.

4. American Hospital Association. Hospital Statistics. Chicago. 1999. See also: Brennan, Troyen A.; Leape, Lucian L.; Laird, Nan M., et al. Incidence of adverse events and negligence in hospitalized patients: Results of the Harvard Medical Practice Study I. *N Engl J Med.* 324:370–376, 1991. See also: Leape, Lucian L.; Brennan, Troyen A.; Laird, Nan M., et al. The Nature of Adverse Events in Hospitalized Patients: Results of the Harvard Medical Practice Study II. *N Engl J Med.* 324(6):377–384, 1991.

5. Centers for Disease Control and Prevention (National Center for Health Statistics). Deaths: Final Data for 1997. *National Vital Statistics Reports.* 47(19):27, 1999.

6. Centers for Disease Control and Prevention (National Center for Health Statistics). Births and Deaths: Preliminary Data for 1998. *National Vital Statistics Reports.* 47(25):6, 1999.

7. Thomas, Eric J.; Studdert, David M.; Newhouse, Joseph P., et al. Costs of Medical Injuries in Utah and Colorado. *Inquiry.* 36:255–264, 1999. See also: Johnson, W.G.;

Brennan, Troyen A.; Newhouse, Joseph P., et al. The Economic Consequences of Medical Injuries. *JAMA*. 267:2487–2492, 1992.

8. Occupational Safety and Health Administration. The New OSHA: Reinventing Worker Safety and Health [Web Page]. Dec. 16, 1998. Available at: www.osha.gov/oshinfo/reinvent.html.

9. Phillips, David P.; Christenfeld, Nicholas; and Glynn, Laura M. Increase in US Medication-Error Deaths between 1983 and 1993. *The Lancet*. 351:643–644, 1998.

10. Bates, David W.; Spell, Nathan; Cullen, David J., et al. The Costs of Adverse Drug Events in Hospitalized Patients. *JAMA*. 277:307–311, 1997.

11. Leape, Lucian; Brennan, Troyen; Laird, Nan; et al., The Nature of Adverse Events in Hospitalized Patients, Results of the Harvard Medical Practice Study II. *N Engl J Med*. 324(6):377–384, 1991.

12. Milstein, Arnold, presentation at "Developing a National Policy Agenda for Improving Patient Safety," meeting sponsored by National Patient Safety Foundation, Joint Commission on Accreditation of Health Care Organizations and American Hospital Association, July 15, 1999, Washington, D.C.

13. Veatch, Robert M., Cross-Cultural Perspectives in Medical Ethics: Readings. Boston: Jones and Bartlett Publishers, 1989.

14. Reason, James T., *Human Error,* Cambridge: Cambridge University Press, 1990.

15. Deming, W. Edwards, *Out of the Crisis*, Cambridge: Massachusetts Institute of Technology, Center for Advanced Engineering Study, 1993.

16. Berwick, Donald M. and Leape, Lucian L. Reducing Errors in Medicine. *BMJ*. 319:136–137, 1999.

17. Brennan, Troyen A.; Leape, Lucian L.; Laird, Nan M, et al. Incidence of Adverse Events and Negligence in Hospitalized Patients. *N Eng J Med*. 324(6):370–376, 1991. See also: Thomas, Eric J.; Studdert, David M.; Newhouse, Joseph P., et al. Costs of Medical Injuries in Utah and Colorado. *Inquiry*. 36:255–264, 1999.

18. Thomas, Eric J.; Studdert, David M.; Newhouse, Joseph P., et al. Costs of Medical Injuries in Utah and Colorado. *Inquiry*. 36:255–264, 1999.

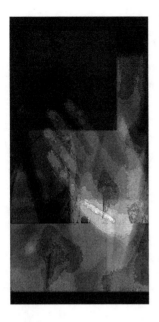

1

A Comprehensive Approach to Improving Patient Safety

This report proposes a comprehensive approach for reducing medical errors and improving patient safety. The approach employs market and regulatory strategies, public and private strategies, and strategies that are implemented inside health care organizations as well as in their external environment. To achieve a threshold improvement in patient safety, all of these strategies must be employed in a balanced and complementary fashion.

This introductory chapter first discusses patient safety within the overall context of improving quality. The objective of the Quality of Health Care in America Project is to lay out a strategy for achieving a threshold improvement in quality over the coming decade. Patient safety is one of three domains of quality concerns. A general model of how the external environment influences health care organizations to improve different domains of quality is presented and the model is then discussed as it applies to patient safety, the focus of this first report of the Quality of Health Care in America Committee. Second, the chapter provides a roadmap to the remainder of the report by briefly describing the chapters that follow.

PATIENT SAFETY:
A CRITICAL COMPONENT OF QUALITY

A general model of the influence of the environment on quality, as shown in Figure 1.1, contains two primary dimensions. The first dimension identifies domains of quality. These include: safe care, practice that is consistent with current medical knowledge and customization. The second dimension identifies forces in the external environment that can drive quality improvement in the delivery system. These have been grouped into two broad categories: regulatory/legislative activities, and economic and other incentives.

Safety, the first domain of quality, refers to "freedom from accidental injury." This definition is stated from the patient's perspective. As discussed in chapter 2 of this report, health care is not as safe as it should be.

The second domain refers to the provision of services in a manner that is consistent with current medical knowledge and best practices. Currently,

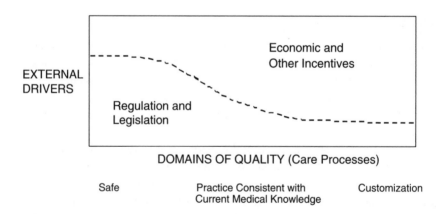

External Drivers: Two categories of factors that can influence quality improvement—regulation and legislation, and economic and other incentives such as actions by purchasers and consumers or professional and community values.

Safe: Freedom from accidental injury. Requires a larger role for regulation and oversight authority.

Practice Consistent with Current Medical Knowledge: Best practices, incorporating evidence-based medicine.

Customization: Meeting customer-specific values and expectations. Requires a larger role for creative, continuous improvement and innovation within organizations and marketplace reward.

FIGURE 1.1 A general model of the influence of the external environment on quality.

there is a great deal of variability in medical practice and, oftentimes, a lack of adherence to medical standards based on scientific evidence.[1]

The third domain exemplifies the ability to meet customer-specific values and expectations, permitting the greatest responsiveness to individual values and preferences and maximum personalization or customization of care. Strong policy directives are difficult to implement in this area because of the variety of individual needs and preferences.

Previous work by the IOM categorized quality problems into misuse (avoidable complications that prevent patients from receiving full potential benefit of a service), overuse (potential for harm from the provision of a service exceeds the possible benefit) and underuse (failure to provide a service that would have produced a favorable outcome for the patient).[2] Within this framework, issues of misuse are most likely to be addressed under safety concerns. Issues of overuse and underuse are most likely to be addressed under the domain of practice consistent with current medical knowledge.

Activities in the external environment are grouped under two general categories: (1) regulation and legislative action and (2) economic and other incentives (or barriers). Regulation and legislation include any form of public policy or legal influence, such as licensing or the liability system. Economic and other incentives constitute a broad category that includes the collective and individual actions of purchasers and consumers, the norms and values of health professionals, and the social values of the nation and local communities.

Regulation and legislative action can influence quality in health care organizations in two ways. First, it can empower the chief executive officer and governance of health care organizations to take action internally to improve quality. It provides a call to action from the external environment that requires a response inside the organization, and lack of an appropriate response generally results in certain sanctions. Second, it requires *all* health care organizations to make minimum investments in systems for quality, thus creating a more level playing field throughout the industry. It should also be noted, however, that regulation and legislation can also create disincentives for quality, such as lax or conflicting standards.

Marketplace incentives direct the values, culture, and priorities of health care organizations and reward performance beyond the minimum. One way this can happen is by purchasers and consumers requesting and using information to direct their business to the best organizations and providers in a community. Both public and private purchasers can be a strong influence, although public purchasers (especially the Health Care Financing Administration) are perceived as a potentially stronger force because of the size of the population they cover as a single purchaser and also because of the additional demands they can bring through conditions of participation and other oversight responsibilities. In health care, efforts to make comparative performance data available in the public domain to assist purchasers and consumers in identifying high quality providers are just starting to emerge through activities such as the Health Plan Employer Data and Information Set (HEDIS) of the National Committee for Quality Assurance (NCQA) and the Consumer Assessment of Health Plans (CAHPs) survey from the Agency for Healthcare Research and Quality (AHRQ).

Although purchasing activities are a major component of the marketplace, health care is not driven by only economic factors. Incentives come from other directions as well, including the norms, values and standards of health professionals and social values of communities. Professional groups, such as medical societies, specialty groups and associations, play a role in defining norms and standards of practice, and setting expectations and values, beginning with training and education and continuing into practice. Such standards and values not only influence the members of a profession, but also the expectations of consumers and others. Additionally, health professionals and health care organizations are expected to respond to social demands, such as caring for the uninsured or working collaboratively to improve health status in local communities. Media, advocacy, and others also influence organizational and professional behavior, but do so indirectly, often working through other parties that have direct influence, such as purchasers and consumers.

Activities in the external environment interact with each other in various ways for the different domains of quality. As noted by the curve in Figure 1.1, the committee believes regulation and legislation play a particularly important role in assuring a basic level of safety for everyone using the health system. Economic, professional and other incentives can, and should, reinforce that priority. On the other hand, the customization of care to meet individual needs and preferences is more driven by economic and other incentives, with regulation and legislation potentially playing a supportive or enabling role. Encouraging practice consistent with current medical knowledge is reflected as a joint responsibility.

The committee believes that a basic level of safety should be assured for all who use the health system and a strong regulatory component is critical to accomplishing this goal. In most industries, ensuring safety is a traditional role of public policy, enforced through regulation. A regulatory authority generally defines minimum levels of capability or expected performance. Through some type of monitoring mechanism (e.g., surveillance system, complaint or reporting system, inspections), problems can be identified and corrective action taken to maintain the minimum levels of performance.

However, the committee recognizes that regulation alone will not be sufficient for achieving a significant improvement in patient safety. Careful alignment of regulatory, economic, professional and other incentives in the external environment is critical if significant improvements in safety are to occur. In developing its recommendations, the committee sought a careful balance between the regulatory/legislative influences and the influence of economic and other incentives. The precise balance that will prove most successful in achieving safety improvements is unknown. Ongoing evaluation should assess whether the proper balance has been achieved relative to safety or if refinement is needed.

The committee's strategy for improving patient safety is for the external environment to create sufficient pressure to make errors so costly in terms of ability to conduct business in the marketplace, market share and reputation that the organization *must* take action. The cost should be high enough that organizations and professionals invest the attention and resources necessary to improve safety. Such external pressures are virtually absent in health care today. The actions of regulatory bodies, group purchasers, consumers and professional groups are all critical to achieving this goal. At the same time, investments in an adequate knowledge base and tools to improve safety are also important to assist health care organizations in responding to this challenge.

ORGANIZATION OF THE REPORT

Following is a brief description of each of the remaining chapters in the report. As a whole, these chapters lay out a rationale for taking strong actions to improve patient safety; a comprehensive strategy for leveraging the actions of regulators, purchasers, consumers, and professionals; and a plan to bolster the knowledge base and tools necessary to improve patient safety.

Chapter 2 of this report, Errors in Health Care: A Leading Cause of Death and Injury, reviews the literature on errors to assess current understanding of the magnitude of the problem and identifies a number of issues that inhibit attention to patient safety. A general lack of information on and awareness of errors in health care by purchasers and consumers makes it impossible for them to demand better care. The culture of medicine creates an expectation of perfection and attributes errors to carelessness or incompetence. Liability concerns discourage the surfacing of errors and communication about how to correct them. The lack of explicit and consistent standards for patient safety creates gaps in licensing and accreditation and lets health care organizations function without some of the basic safety systems in place. The lack of any agency or organization with primary responsibility for patient safety prevents the dissemination of any cohesive message about patient safety. Given the gaps in the external environment, it should come as no surprise that the health care delivery system is not as responsive as it could be to concerns about patient safety. The external environment is not creating any requirement or demand for the delivery system to reduce medical errors and improve the safety of patients.

Chapter 3, Why Do Errors Happen?, offers a discussion of several concepts in patient safety, including a number of definitions for terms used throughout this report. The chapter describes leading theory on why accidents happen and the types of errors that occur. It also explores why some systems are safer than others and the contribution of human factors principles to designing safer systems.

Chapters 4 through 8 of the report lay out a set of actions that the external environment can take to increase attention by the delivery system to issues of patient safety. They also identify a set of actions that the delivery system can pursue in response. The combination of proposed strategies seeks to build a national focus on patient safety, make more and better information available, set explicit standards for patient safety, and identify how health care organizations can put safety systems into practice.

Chapter 4, Building Leadership and Knowledge to Improve Patient Safety, discusses the need for a focal point for patient safety. The lack of a clear focal point makes it difficult to define priorities, call for action where needed, or produce a consistent message about safety. Other high-risk industries can identify an agency or organization with accountability for monitoring and communicating about safety problems. No such focal point exists in health care. The chapter discusses the role of national leadership to set aims and to track progress over time in achieving these aims, the need to develop and fund a safety agenda, and approaches for improving dissemination and outreach about safety to the marketplace and to regulators and policy makers.

Chapter 5, Error Reporting Systems, discusses reporting systems as one means for obtaining information about medical errors. A number of public and private reporting systems currently exist, some focused on very specific issues, such as medications, and others are more broad based. However, collecting reports on errors is only part of the picture. Analyzing and using the information is how improvements can occur. This chapter discusses the role and purpose of error reporting systems, how to maximize the availability and use of reports, and the contribution of existing reporting systems.

Chapter 6, Protecting Voluntary Error Reporting Systems from Legal Discovery, identifies the legal constraints on protecting data submitted to voluntary reporting systems. Health care organizations are concerned that sharing information about medical errors will expose them to litigation. The unwillingness to share such information means that errors remain hidden and the same errors may be repeated in different organizations. The chapter discusses the legal and practical options available for protecting data to let providers and health care organizations more openly discuss issues related to medical error and patient safety so that errors can be prevented before they result in serious harm or death.

Chapter 7, Setting Performance Standards and Expectations for Safety, discusses the need for explicit and consistent standards for patient safety. Such standards not only define minimum expected levels of performance, but also set expectations for purchasers and consumers. The roles of licensing and accrediting bodies are discussed relative to standards for health care organizations, professionals, and drugs and medical devices. The roles of purchasers and professional groups in setting expectations are also discussed.

Chapter 8, Creating Safety Systems in Health Care Organizations, discusses actions within the delivery system to improve patient safety. The goal for improving patient safety is to affect the delivery of care. Health care organizations have to make certain that systems are in place to ensure patient safety, but they also have to build in mechanisms for learning about safety concerns and for continuous improvement. The chapter discusses the importance of an organizational commitment to safety and the need to incorporate safety principles into operational processes.

Before proceeding further, it is useful to identify what this report is *not*. Three distinct issues that have been raised during various discussions on patient safety are not addressed here. First, the committee recognizes that a major force for improving patient safety is intrinsic motivation, that is, it is driven by the values and attitudes of health professionals and health care organizations. This report, however, focuses primarily on the external environment and the policy and market strategies that can be employed to encourage actions by health professionals and health care organizations. It is hoped that actions in the external environment will lead to implementation of a specific set of actions within health care organizations. Although some health care organizations are already implementing the recommended actions absent any incentives from the external environment, the external environment can motivate a broader response.

Second, worker safety is often linked with patient safety. If workers are safer in their jobs, patients will be safer also. Sometimes, the actions needed to improve patient safety are ones that would also improve worker safety. Procedures for avoiding needlesticks or limiting long work hours are aimed at protecting workers but can also protect patients. Thus, although worker safety is not the focus of this report, the committee believes that creating a safe environment for patients will go a long way in addressing issues of worker safety as well.

The third issue is that of access to care. This report is focused on making the delivery of care safer for patients who have access to and are using the health care system. Safe care is an important part of quality care. Although safe care does not guarantee quality, it is a necessary prerequisite for the delivery of high-quality care. However, the committee also recognizes the relationship that exists between access and quality. When someone needs medical care, the worst quality is no care at all.

Access continues to be threatened in today's health care marketplace. For many people the lack of insurance creates a significant barrier to access. The uninsured typically use fewer services than the insured, are more likely to report having cost and access problems, and are less likely to believe that they receive excellent care.[3] However, access is not just a concern of the uninsured. Even people with insurance are growing uneasy about their access to care. Employers are reducing coverage for workers and their dependents.[4] Inadequate coverage compromises access and creates inequities between those who have complete coverage and full access and those who have partial coverage and partial access. Insufficient coverage also creates concerns about the affordability of care, either because services are not covered at all or because significant out-of-pocket payments, such as copayments and deductibles, are involved. Although financial burden is a significant barrier to access, other factors interfere as well, such as poor transportation, language, and cultural barriers.[5]

When access to care is threatened, the ability to make a threshold change in quality is also threatened. Although it is not being addressed in this report, those dealing with overall quality concerns will also have to consider problems of access.

REFERENCES

1. Chassin, Mark R.; Galvin, Robert W.; and the National Roundtable on Health Care Quality. The Urgent Need to Improve Health Care Quality. *JAMA.* 280(11):1000–1005, 1998. See also: Advisory Commission on Consumer Protection and Quality in the Health Care Industry. Quality First: Better Health Care for All Americans. U.S. Department of Health and Human Services. 1998.

2. Chassin, Mark R.; Galvin, Robert W.; and the National Roundtable on Health Care Quality. The Urgent Need to Improve Health Care Quality. *JAMA.* 280(11):1000–1005, 1998.

3. Berk, Marc L., and Schur, Claudia L. Measuring Access to Care: Improving Information for Policymakers. *Health Affairs.* 17(1):180–186, 1998. Also, Donelan, Karen; Blendon, Robert J.; Schoen, Cathy, et al. The Cost of Health System Change: Public Discontent in Five Nations. *Health Affairs.* 18(3):206–216, 1999.

4. Kronick, Richard, and Gilmer, Todd. Explaining the Decline in Health Insurance Coverage, 1979–1995. *Health Affairs.* 18(2):30–47, 1999.

5. Institute of Medicine. *Access to Health Care in America.* Michael Millman, ed. Washington, D.C.: National Academy Press, 1993.

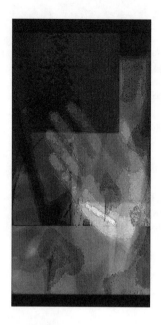

2
Errors in Health Care: A Leading Cause of Death and Injury

Health care is not as safe as it should be. A substantial body of evidence points to medical errors as a leading cause of death and injury.

• Sizable numbers of Americans are harmed as a result of medical errors. Two studies of large samples of hospital admissions, one in New York using 1984 data and another in Colorado and Utah using 1992 data, found that the proportion of hospital admissions experiencing an adverse event, defined as injuries caused by medical management, were 2.9 and 3.7 percent,[1] respectively. The proportion of adverse events attributable to errors (i.e., preventable adverse events) was 58 percent in New York, and 53 percent in Colorado and Utah.[2]

• Preventable adverse events are a leading cause of death in the United States. When extrapolated to the over 33.6 million admissions to U.S. hospitals in 1997, the results of these two studies imply that at least 44,000 and perhaps as many as 98,000 Americans die in hospitals each year as a result of medical errors.[3] Even when using the lower estimate, deaths in hospitals due to preventable adverse events exceed the number attributable to the 8th-leading cause of death.[4] Deaths due to preventable adverse events exceed the deaths attributable to motor vehicle accidents (43,458), breast cancer (42,297) or AIDS (16,516).[5]

- Total national costs (lost income, lost household production, disability, health care costs) are estimated to be between $37.6 billion and $50 · billion for adverse events and between $17 billion and $29 billion for preventable adverse events.[6] Health care costs account for over one-half of the total costs. Even when using the lower estimates, the total national costs associated with adverse events and preventable adverse events represent approximately 4 percent and 2 percent, respectively, of national health expenditures in 1996.[7] In 1992, the direct and indirect costs of adverse events were slightly higher than the direct and indirect costs of caring for people with HIV and AIDS.[8]

- In terms of lives lost, patient safety is as important an issue as worker safety. Although more than 6,000 Americans die from workplace injuries every year,[9,10] in 1993 medication errors are estimated to have accounted for about 7,000 deaths.[11] Medication errors account for one out of 131 outpatient deaths and one out of 854 inpatient deaths.

- Medication-related errors occur frequently in hospitals; not all result in actual harm, but those that do are costly. One recent study conducted at two prestigious teaching hospitals found that almost two percent of admissions experienced a preventable adverse drug event, resulting in average increased hospital costs of $4,700 per admission or about $2.8 million annually for a 700-bed teaching hospital.[12] If these findings are generalizable, the increased hospital costs alone of preventable adverse drug events affecting inpatients are about $2 billion for the nation as a whole.

- Hospital patients represent only a fraction of the total population at risk of experiencing a medication-related error. In 1998, nearly 2.5 billion prescriptions were dispensed by U.S. pharmacies at a cost of about $92 billion.[13] Numerous studies document errors in prescribing medications,[14,15] dispensing by pharmacists,[16] and unintentional nonadherence on the part of the patient.[17] Medication errors have the potential to increase as a major contributor to avoidable morbidity and mortality as new medications are introduced for a wider range of indications.

This chapter provides a summary of findings in the literature on the frequency and cost of health care errors and the factors that contribute to their occurrence.

INTRODUCTION

Although the literature pertaining to errors in health care has grown steadily over the last decade and some notable studies are particularly strong methodologically, we do not yet have a complete picture of the epidemiology of errors. Many studies focus on patients experiencing injury and provide valuable insight into the magnitude of harm resulting from errors. Other studies, more limited in number, focus on the occurrence of errors, both those that result in harm and those that do not (sometimes called "near misses"). More is known about errors that occur in hospitals than in other health care delivery settings.

Synthesizing and interpreting the findings in the literature pertaining to errors in health care is complicated due to the absence of standardized nomenclature. For purposes of this report, the terms error and adverse event are defined as follows:

An error is defined as the failure of a planned action to be completed as intended (i.e., error of execution) or the use of a wrong plan to achieve an aim (i.e., error of planning).[18]

An adverse event is an injury caused by medical management rather than the underlying condition of the patient. An adverse event attributable to error is a "preventable adverse event."[19] *Negligent adverse events represent a subset of preventable adverse events that satisfy legal criteria used in determining negligence (i.e., whether the care provided failed to meet the standard of care reasonably expected of an average physician qualified to take care of the patient in question).*[20]

When a study in the literature has used a definition that deviates from the above definitions, it is noted below.

Medication-related error has been studied extensively for several reasons: it is one of the most common types of error, substantial numbers of individuals are affected, and it accounts for a sizable increase in health care costs.[21–23] There are also methodologic issues: (1) prescription drugs are widely used, so it is easy to identify an adequate sample of patients who experience adverse drug events; (2) the drug prescribing process provides good documentation of medical decisions, and much of this documentation resides in automated, easily accessible databases; and (3) deaths attributable to medication errors are recorded on death certificates. There are probably other areas of health care delivery that have been studied to a lesser degree but may offer equal or greater opportunity for improvement in safety.

Efforts to assess the importance of various types of errors are currently hampered by the lack of a standardized taxonomy for reporting adverse events, errors, and risk factors.[24,25] A limited number of studies focus directly on the causes of adverse events, but attempts to classify adverse events according to "root causes" are complicated by the fact that several interlocking factors often contribute to an error or series of errors that in turn result in an adverse event.[26,27] In recent years, some progress toward a more standardized nomenclature and taxonomy has been made in the medication area, but much work remains to be done.[28]

The following discussion of the literature addresses four questions:

1. How frequently do errors occur?
2. What factors contribute to errors?
3. What are the costs of errors?
4. Are public perceptions of safety in health care consistent with the evidence?

HOW FREQUENTLY DO ERRORS OCCUR?

For the most part, studies that provide insight into the incidence and prevalence of errors fall into two categories:

1. *General studies of patients experiencing adverse events.* These are studies of adverse events in general, not studies limited to medication-related events. These studies are limited in number, but some represent large-scale, multi-institutional analyses. Virtually all studies in this category focus on hospitalized patients. With the exception of medication-related events discussed in the second category, little if any research has focused on errors or adverse events occurring outside of hospital settings, for example, in ambulatory care clinics, surgicenters, office practices, home health, or care administered by patients, their family, and friends at home.

2. *Studies of patients experiencing medication-related errors.* There is an abundance of studies that fall into this category. Although many focus on errors and adverse events associated with ordering and administering medication to hospitalized patients, some studies focus on patients in ambulatory settings.

Adverse Events

An adverse event is defined as an injury caused by medical management rather than by the underlying disease or condition of the patient.[29] Not all, but a sizable proportion of adverse events are the result of errors. Numerous studies have looked at the proportion of adverse events attributable to medical error. Due to methodologic challenges, far fewer studies focus on the full range of error—namely, those that result in injury *and* those that expose the patient to risk but do not result in injury.

The most extensive study of adverse events is the Harvard Medical Practice Study, a study of more than 30,000 randomly selected discharges from 51 randomly selected hospitals in New York State in 1984.[30] Adverse events, manifest by prolonged hospitalization or disability at the time of discharge or both, occurred in 3.7 percent of the hospitalizations. The proportion of adverse events attributable to errors (i.e., preventable adverse events) was 58 percent and the proportion of adverse events due to negligence was 27.6 percent. Although most of these adverse events gave rise to disability lasting less than six months, 13.6 percent resulted in death and 2.6 percent caused permanently disabling injuries. Drug complications were the most common type of adverse event (19 percent), followed by wound infections (14 percent) and technical complications (13 percent).[31,32]

The findings of the Harvard Medical Practice Study in New York have recently been corroborated by a study of adverse events in Colorado and Utah occurring in 1992.[33] This study included the review of medical records pertaining to a random sample of 15,000 discharges from a representative sample of hospitals in the two states. Adverse events occurred in 2.9 percent of hospitalizations in each state. Over four out of five of these adverse events occurred in the hospital, the remaining occurred prior to admission in physicians' offices, patients' homes or other non-hospital settings. The proportion of adverse events due to negligence was 29.2 percent, and the proportion of adverse events that were preventable was 53 percent.[34] As was the case in the New York study, over 50 percent of adverse events were minor, temporary injuries. But the study in New York found that 13.6 percent of adverse events led to death, as compared with 6.6 percent in Colorado and Utah. In New York, about one in four negligent adverse events led to death, while in Colorado and Utah, death resulted in about 1 out of every 11 negligent adverse events. Factors that might explain the differences between the two studies include: temporal changes in health care, and differences in the states' patient populations and health care systems.[35]

Both the study in New York and the study in Colorado and Utah identified a subset of preventable adverse events that also satisfied criteria applied by the legal system in determining negligence. It is important to note that although some of these cases may stem from incompetent or impaired providers, the committee believes that many could likely have been avoided had better systems of care been in place.

Extrapolation of the results of the Colorado and Utah study to the over 33.6 million admissions to hospitals in the United States in 1997, implies that at least 44,000 Americans die in hospitals each year as a result of preventable medical errors.[36] Based on the results of the New York study, the number of deaths due to medical error may be as high as 98,000.[37] By way of comparison, the lower estimate is greater than the number of deaths attributable to the 8th-leading cause of death.[38]

Some maintain these extrapolations likely underestimate the occurrence of preventable adverse events because these studies: (1) considered only those patients whose injuries resulted in a specified level of harm; (2) imposed a high threshold to determine whether an adverse event was preventable or negligent (concurrence of two reviewers); and (3) included only errors that are documented in patient records.[39]

Two studies that relied on both medical record abstraction and other information sources, such as provider reports, have found higher rates of adverse events occurring in hospitals. In a study of 815 consecutive patients on a general medical service of a university hospital, it was found that 36 percent had an iatrogenic illness, defined as any illness that resulted from a diagnostic procedure, from any form of therapy, or from a harmful occurrence that was not a natural consequence of the patient's disease.[40] Of the 815 patients, nine percent had an iatrogenic illness that threatened life or produced considerable disability, and for another two percent, iatrogenic illness was believed to contribute to the death of the patient.

In a study of 1,047 patients admitted to two intensive care units and one surgical unit at a large teaching hospital, 480 (45.8 percent) were identified as having had an adverse event, where adverse event was defined as "situations in which an inappropriate decision was made when, at the time, an appropriate alternative could have been chosen."[41] For 185 patients (17.7 percent), the adverse event was serious, producing disability or death. The likelihood of experiencing an adverse event increased about six percent for each day of hospital stay.

Some information on errors can also be gleaned from studies that focus on inpatients who died or experienced a myocardial infarction or postsurgical complication. In a study of 182 deaths in 12 hospitals from three conditions (cerebrovascular accident, pneumonia, or myocardial infarction), it was found that at least 14 percent and possibly as many as 27 percent of the deaths might have been prevented.[42] A 1991 analysis of 203 incidents of cardiac arrest at a teaching hospital,[43] found that 14 percent followed an iatrogenic complication and that more than half of these might have been prevented. In a study of 44,603 patients who underwent surgery between

1977 and 1990 at a large medical center, 2,428 patients (5.4 percent) suffered complications and nearly one-half of these complications were attributable to error.[44] Another 749 died during the same hospitalization; 7.5 percent of these deaths were attributed to error.

Patients who died during surgery requiring general anesthesia have been the focus of many studies over the last few decades. Anesthesia is an area in which very impressive improvements in safety have been made. As more and more attention has been focused on understanding the factors that contribute to error and on the design of safer systems, preventable mishaps have declined.[45–48] Studies, some conducted in Australia, the United Kingdom and other countries, indicate that, today, anesthesia mortality rates are about one death per 200,000–300,000 anesthetics administered, compared with two deaths per 10,000 anesthetics in the early 1980s.[49] The gains in anesthesia are very impressive and were accomplished through a variety of mechanisms, including improved monitoring techniques, the development and widespread adoption of practice guidelines, and other systematic approaches to reducing errors.[50]

Lastly, some studies have relied on incident reporting systems to identify and analyze errors. For example, in Australia, 324 general practitioners participating voluntarily in an incident reporting system reported a total of 805 incidents during October 1993 through June 1995, of which 76 percent were preventable and 27 percent had the potential for severe harm.[51] These studies provide information on the types of errors that occur but are not useful for estimating the incidence of errors, because the population at risk (i.e., the denominator) is generally unknown.

Medication-Related Errors

Even though medication errors that result in death or serious injury occur infrequently, sizable and increasing numbers of people are affected because of the extensive use of drugs in both out-of-hospital and in-hospital settings. In 1998, nearly 2.5 billion prescriptions were dispensed in U.S. pharmacies at an estimated cost of about $92 billion.[52] An estimated 3.75 billion drug administrations were made to patients in hospitals.[53]

In a review of U.S. death certificates between 1983 and 1993, it was found that 7,391 people died in 1993 from medication errors (accidental poisoning by drugs, medicaments, and biologicals that resulted from acknowledged errors by patients or medical personnel), compared with 2,876 people in 1983, representing a 2.57-fold increase.[54] Outpatient deaths due to medication errors rose 8.48-fold during the 10-year period, compared with a 2.37-fold increase in inpatient deaths.

Medication Errors in Hospitals

Medication errors occur frequently in hospitals. Numerous studies have assessed the incidence of adverse drug events (ADEs), defined as an injury resulting from medical intervention related to a drug.[55] Not all ADEs are attributable to errors. For example, a patient with no history of allergic reactions to drugs, who experiences an allergic reaction to an antibiotic, has suffered an ADE, but this ADE would not be attributable to error. However, an error would have occurred if an antibiotic was prescribed to a patient with a history of documented allergic reactions, because the medical record was unavailable or not consulted. We discuss only those studies of ADEs that identified the subset of ADEs determined to be preventable (i.e., attributable to errors).

In an analysis of 289,411 medication orders written during one year in a tertiary-care teaching hospital, the overall error rate was estimated to be 3.13 errors for each 1,000 orders written and the rate of significant errors to be 1.81 per 1,000 orders.[56] In a review of 4,031 adult admissions to 11 medical and surgical units at two tertiary care hospitals, Bates et al. identified 247 ADEs for an extrapolated event rate of 6.5 ADEs per 100 nonobstetrical admissions, and a mean number per hospital per year of approximately 1,900 ADEs.[57] Twenty-eight percent were judged preventable.

In a study of patients admitted to coronary intensive care, medical, surgical, and obstetric units in an urban tertiary care hospital over a 37-day period, the rate of drug-related incidents was 73 in 2,967 patient-days: 27 incidents were judged ADEs; 34, potential ADEs; and 12, problem orders.[58] Of the 27 ADEs, five were life threatening, nine were serious, and 13 were significant. Of the 27 ADEs, 15(56 percent) were judged definitely or probably preventable. In a study of prescribing errors detected and averted by pharmacists in a 631-bed tertiary care teaching hospital between July 1994 and June 1995, the estimated overall rate of errors was 3.99 per 1,000 medication orders.[59]

Children are at particular risk of medication errors, and as discussed below, this is attributable primarily to incorrect dosages.[60,61] In a study of 101,022 medication orders at two children's teaching hospitals, a total of 479 errant medication orders were identified, of which 27 represented potentially lethal prescribing errors.[62] The frequency of errors was similar at the two institutions, 4.9 and 4.5 errors per 1,000 medication orders. The error rate per 100 patient-days was greater in the pediatric intensive care units (PICUs) than in the pediatric ward or neonatal intensive care units, and the authors attribute this to the greater heterogeneity of patients cared for in PICUs and the broad range of drugs and dosages used. In a four-year prospective quality assurance study, 315 medication errors resulting in injury were reported among the 2,147 neonatal and pediatric intensive care admissions, an error rate of one per 6.8 admissions.[63] The frequency of iatrogenic injury of any sort due to a medication error was 3.1 percent—one injury for each 33 intensive care admissions.

Not surprisingly, the potential for medication-related error increases as the average number of drugs administered increases. In a prospective cohort study of 4,031 adult admissions to 11 medical and surgical units in two tertiary care hospitals (including two medical and three surgical ICUs), the rate of preventable ADEs and preventable potential ADEs in ICUs was 19 events per 1,000 patient-days, nearly twice the rate of non-ICUs.[64] When adjusted for the number of drugs used in the previous 24 hours or ordered since admission, there were no differences in error rates between ICUs and non-ICUs.

Current estimates of the incidence of medication errors are undoubtedly low because many errors go undocumented and unreported.[65-68] For example, in a study of patients admitted to five patient care units at a tertiary care hospital during a six month period in 1993, it was found that incident reports were filed with the hospital's quality assurance program or called into the pharmacy hotline for only three of the 54 people experiencing an adverse drug event.[69]

Some errors are also difficult to detect in the absence of computerized surveillance systems. In a study of 36,653 hospitalized patients, Classen et al. identified 731 ADEs in 648 patients, but only 92 of these were reported by physicians, pharmacists, and nurses.[70] The remaining 631 were detected from automated signals, the most common of which were diphenhydramine hydrochloride and naloxone hydrochloride use, high serum drug levels, leukopenia, and the use of phytonadione and antidiarrheals.

Medication Errors in Ambulatory Settings

There is evidence indicating that ADEs account for a sizable number of admissions to inpatient facilities, but we do not know what proportion of these ADE-related admissions are attributable to errors. One study found that between three and 11 percent of hospital admissions were attributable to ADEs.[71] A review of 14 Australian studies published between 1988 and 1996 reported that 2.4 to 3.6 percent of all hospital admissions were drug related, and between 32 and 69 percent were definitely or possibly preventable. Drug groups most commonly involved were cytotoxics, cardiovascular agents, antihypertensives, anticoagulants, and nonsteroidal anti-inflammatory drugs.[72]

ADEs also result in increased visits to physician offices and emergency departments. In an analysis of 1,000 patients drawn from a community office-based medical practice who were observed for adverse drug reactions, adverse effects were recorded in 42 (4.2 percent), of which 23 were judged to be unnecessary and potentially avoidable.[73] In an analysis of 62,216 visits to an emergency department by patients enrolled in a health maintenance organization (HMO), it was found that 1,074 (1.7 percent) were related to medication noncompliance or inappropriate prescribing.[74]

There is a sizable body of literature to document the incidence of patient noncompliance with medication regimens, but less is known about the proportion of noncompliance attributable to medical error (defined as accidental or unintentional nonadherence to a therapeutic program) as opposed to intentional noncompliance. In a meta-analysis of seven studies, Sullivan et al. estimate that 5.5 percent of admissions can be attributed to drug therapy noncompliance, amounting to 1.94 million admissions and $8.5 billion in hospital expenditures in 1986.[75] Similar results were obtained by Einarson in a meta-analysis of 37 studies published between 1966 and 1989, which found that hospital admissions caused by ADEs, resulting from noncompliance or unintentionally inappropriate drug use, ranged from 0.2 to 21.7 percent with a median of 4.9 percent and a mean of 5.5 percent.[76] Patient noncompliance is clearly an important quality issue, but it should be emphasized that we do not know the extent to which noncompliance is related to errors.

FACTORS THAT CONTRIBUTE TO ERRORS

Studies of Adverse Events

Patient safety problems of many kinds occur during the course of providing health care. They include transfusion errors and adverse drug events; wrong-site surgery and surgical injuries; preventable suicides; restraint-related injuries or death; hospital-acquired or other treatment-related infections; and falls, burns, pressure ulcers, and mistaken identity. Leape et al.

have characterized the kinds of errors that resulted in medical injury in the Medical Practice Study as diagnostic, treatment, preventive, or other errors (see Box 2.1).

More than two-thirds (70 percent) of the adverse events found in this study were thought to be preventable, with the most common types of preventable errors being technical errors (44 percent), diagnosis (17 percent), failure to prevent injury (12 percent) and errors in the use of a drug (10 percent). The contributions of complexity and technology to such error rates is highlighted by the higher rates of events that occur in the highly technical surgical specialties of vascular surgery, cardiac surgery, and neurosurgery. In hospitals, high error rates with serious consequences are most likely in intensive care units, operating rooms and emergency departments.

Thomas et al., in their study of admissions to hospitals in Colorado and Utah experiencing adverse events, found that about 30 percent were attributable to negligence.[77] The hospital location with the highest proportion of

---

BOX 2.1
Types of Errors

Diagnostic
　　Error or delay in diagnosis
　　Failure to employ indicated tests
　　Use of outmoded tests or therapy
　　Failure to act on results of monitoring or testing

Treatment
　　Error in the performance of an operation, procedure, or test
　　Error in administering the treatment
　　Error in the dose or method of using a drug
　　Avoidable delay in treatment or in responding to an abnormal test
　　Inappropriate (not indicated) care

Preventive
　　Failure to provide prophylactic treatment
　　Inadequate monitoring or follow-up of treatment

Other
　　Failure of communication
　　Equipment failure
　　Other system failure

SOURCE: Leape, Lucian; Lawthers, Ann G.; Brennan, Troyen A., et al. Preventing Medical Injury. *Qual Rev Bull.* 19(5):144–149, 1993.

negligent adverse events (52.6 percent) was the emergency department. The authors note the complexity inherent in emergency medical care and point to the need to improve teamwork and standardize work procedures.

Other studies have made similar attempts to classify errors. Dubois and Brook studied 49 preventable deaths from 12 hospitals, and found that for those who died of a myocardial infarction, preventable deaths reflected errors in management; for cerebrovascular accident, most deaths reflected errors in diagnosis; and for pneumonia, some deaths reflected errors in management and some reflected errors in diagnosis.[78] In an analysis of 203 cardiac arrests at a teaching hospital, Bedell et al. found that of the half that might have been prevented, the most common causes of potentially preventable arrest were medication errors and toxic effects, and suboptimal response by physicians to clinical signs and symptoms.[79]

Studies of Medication Errors

Ensuring appropriate medication use is a complex process involving multiple organizations and professionals from various disciplines; knowledge of drugs; timely access to accurate and complete patient information; and a series of interrelated decisions over a period of time. As shown in Box 2.2, errors can creep into this process at various points. Some errors are errors of commission (e.g., administration of improper drug), while others are errors of omission (e.g., failure to administer a drug that was prescribed).

Medication errors are often preventable, although reducing the error rate significantly will require multiple interventions. In the study of prescribing errors conducted by Lesar et al.,[80] the most common factors associated with errors were decline in renal or hepatic function requiring alteration of drug therapy (13.9 percent); patient history of allergy to the same medication class (12.1 percent); using the wrong drug name, dosage form, or abbreviation (11.4 percent for both brand name and generic name orders); incorrect dosage calculations (11.1 percent); and atypical or unusual and critical dosage frequency considerations (10.8 percent). The most common groups of factors associated with errors were those related to knowledge and the application of knowledge regarding drug therapy (30 percent); knowledge and use of knowledge regarding patient factors that affect drug therapy (29.2 percent); use of calculations, decimal points, or unit and rate expression factors (17.5 percent); and nomenclature—for example incorrect drug name, dosage form, or abbreviations (13.4 percent).

Many studies have identified inappropriate prescribing as a particu-

---

BOX 2.2
Medication Use Processes

Prescribing
- Assessing the need for and selecting the correct drug
- Individualizing the therapeutic regimen
- Designating the desired therapeutic response

Dispensing
- Reviewing the order
- Processing the order
- Compounding and preparing the drug
- Dispensing the drug in a timely manner

Administering
- Administering the right medication to the right patient
- Administering medication when indicated
- Informing the patient about the medication
- Including the patient in administration

Monitoring
- Monitoring and documenting patient's response
- Identifying and reporting adverse drug events
- Reevaluating drug selection, regimen, frequency and duration

Systems and Management Control
- Collaborating and communicating amongst caregivers
- Reviewing and managing patient's complete therapeutic drug regimen

---

SOURCE: Nadzam, Deborah M., Development of medication-use indicators by the Joint Commission on Accreditation of Healthcare Organizations. *AJHP.* 48:1925–1930, 1991.

---

larly important factor in accounting for medication errors. In an analysis of 1987 National Medical Expenditure Survey data, it was found that physicians prescribe potentially inappropriate medications for nearly a quarter of all older people living in the community.[81] In a study of 366 consecutive patients admitted to a department of cardiology, "definite" or "probable" drug events (i.e., adverse drug reactions and dose-related therapeutic failures) accounted for 15 admissions, of which five were judged to be due to error in prescription and another five judged to have been avoidable had appropriate measures been taken by prescribing physicians.[82] In an analysis of 682 children admitted to a Congenital Heart Disease Center at a teaching hospital in the United Kingdom, 441 medication errors were reported by nurses, doctors, and pharmacists, of which prescribing errors accounted for 68 percent, followed by administration errors (25 percent) and supply errors (seven percent).[83] In Burnum's[84] analysis of 1,000 patients drawn from a community office-based medical practice who experienced adverse drug reactions, 23 patients were judged to have experienced an "unnecessary and potentially avoidable" event, 10 of which were due to physician error (i.e., six due to administration of a drug not indicated and four to improper drug administration).

Physicians do not routinely screen for potential drug interactions, even when medication history information is readily available. In an analysis of 424 randomly selected visits to a hospital emergency department, 47 percent led to added medication, and in 10 percent of the visits in which at least one medication was added, the new medication added a potential adverse interaction.[85] In all cases, a medication history was recorded on the patients and available to the physicians.

Errors can occur in the dispensing of drugs by pharmacists. In a recent investigation of pharmacists, the Massachusetts State Board of Registration in Pharmacy estimated that 2.4 million prescriptions are filled improperly each year in Massachusetts.[86] Eighty-eight percent of the errors involved giving patients the wrong drug or the wrong strength.

Errors in the ordering and administration of medications are common in hospitals. Bates et al.,[87] in an analysis of more than 4,000 admissions to two tertiary care hospitals, found that about 28 percent of 247 adverse drug events were preventable and most of these resulted from errors that occurred at the stages of ordering and administration. Davis and Cohen[88] in their review of the literature and other evidence on errors report an error rate of 12 percent to be common in the preparation and administration of medications in hospitals. In a study of medication orders at two children's teaching hospitals, Folli et al.[89] found that errors occurred in almost five out of every 1,000 orders and that the most prevalent error was overdose.

Patients make errors too. With greater emphasis on community-based long-term care, increased ambulatory surgery, shorter hospital lengths of stay, and greater reliance on complex drug therapy, patients play an increasingly important role in the administration of drugs. Greenberg et al.[90] found that 4.3 percent of the elderly enrolled in Medicare social HMOs required assistance with the administration of medications. The inability to manage complex drug therapies explains why some elderly are in institutional rather than community-based long-term-care settings.[91]

Automated information and decision support systems are effective in reducing many types of errors. In an analysis of admissions to 11 medical and surgical units at two tertiary care hospitals, Leape et al.[92] identified 334 errors as the causes of 264 preventable ADEs and potential ADEs. About three out of four errors were caused by one of seven types of systems failures (drug knowledge dissemination, dose and identity checking, patient information availability, order transcription, allergy defense, medication order tracking, and interservice communication), and all could have been improved by better information systems that disseminate knowledge about drugs and make drug and patient information readily accessible at the time it is needed.

Computerized drug order entry systems have much potential to reduce errors. In a study of 379 consecutive admissions to three medical units at an urban tertiary care hospital, 10,070 medication orders were written and 530 medication errors were identified (5.3 errors per 100 orders). More than half of the medication errors involved at least one missing dose of a medication.[93] Of the 530 medication errors, five (0.9 percent) resulted in adverse drug events that were judged preventable, and another 35 represented potential adverse drug events (i.e., medication errors with the potential for injury but in which no injury occurred). Physician computer order entry could have prevented 84 percent missing dose medication errors, 86 percent of potential adverse drug events, and 60 percent of preventable adverse drug events. However, more sophisticated technology is not the only option; involving pharmacists in reviewing drug orders significantly reduced the potential harm resulting from errant medication orders.[94,95]

THE COST OF ERRORS

In addition to the unfortunate health consequences suffered by many as a result of medical error, there are direct and indirect costs borne by society as a whole as a result of medical errors. Direct costs refer to higher health care expenditures, while indirect costs include factors such as lost productivity, disability costs, and personal costs of care.

Based on analysis of 459 adverse events identified by reviewing the medical records of 14,732 randomly selected 1992 discharges from 28 hospitals in Colorado and Utah, Thomas et al. estimated the total costs (lost income, lost household production, disability and health care costs) to be nearly $662 million of which health care costs totaled $348 million.[96] The total costs associated with the 265 of the 459 adverse events that were found to be preventable were $308 million, of which $159 million represented health care costs. Based on extrapolation to all hospital admissions in the United

States, the authors estimate the national costs of adverse events to be $37.6 billion and of preventable adverse events to be $17 billion. The total national costs associated with adverse events was approximately 4 percent of national health expenditures in 1996. In 1992, the direct and indirect costs of adverse events were slightly higher than the direct and indirect costs of caring for people with HIV and AIDS.

It has been estimated that for every dollar spent on ambulatory medications, another dollar is spent to treat new health problems caused by the medication.[97] Studies of the direct costs of medication-related errors fall into three categories; (1) population-based studies of patients in a community or health plan; (2) studies of medication-related errors that occur in hospitals; and (3) studies of medication-related errors that occur in nursing homes.

One estimate places the annual national health care cost of drug-related morbidity and mortality in the ambulatory setting as high as $76.6 billion in 1994.[98] Not all drug-related morbidity and mortality is preventable, but numerous studies document errors in prescribing,[99,100] dispensing by pharmacists,[101] and unintentional nonadherence on the part of the patient.[102]

Medication-related errors occur frequently, most do not result in actual harm, but those that do are costly. One recent study conducted at two prestigious teaching hospitals found that almost two percent of admissions experienced a preventable ADE, resulting in an average increased length of stay of 4.6 days and an average increased hospital cost of nearly $4,700 per admission.[103] This amounts to about $2.8 million annually for a 700-bed teaching hospital, and if these findings are generalizable, the increased hospital costs alone of preventable adverse drug events affecting inpatients are about $2 billion for the nation as a whole.

In a matched case-control study of all patients admitted to a large teaching hospital from January 1990 through December 1993, it was found that adverse drug events complicated 2.43 admissions per 100.[104] Controls were matched to cases on primary discharge diagnosis related group (DRG), age, sex, acuity, and year of admission. The occurrence of an ADE was associated with an increased length of stay of 1.91 days and an increased cost of $2,262. The increased risk of death among patients experiencing an adverse drug event was 1.88.

Other studies corroborate the high cost of medication-related errors. One study conducted in a university-affiliated medical center hospital estimated that the annual costs of treating the 1,911 medication-related problems identified through the hospital's voluntary reporting system in 1994 totaled slightly less than $1.5 million.[105] Bloom has estimated that $3.9 billion was spent in 1983 to manage the preventable gastrointestinal adverse effects of nonsteroidal anti-inflammatory drugs.[106]

Medication-related errors also occur in nursing homes. For every dollar spent on drugs in nursing facilities, $1.33 is consumed in the treatment of drug-related morbidity and mortality, amounting to $7.6 billion for the nation as a whole, of which $3.6 billion has been estimated to be avoidable.[107]

PUBLIC PERCEPTIONS OF SAFETY

Although the risk of dying as a result of a medical error far surpasses the risk of dying in an airline accident, a good deal more public attention has been focused on improving safety in the airline industry than in the health care industry. The likelihood of dying per domestic jet flight is estimated to be one in eight million.[108] Statistically, an average passenger would have to fly around the clock for more than 438 years before being involved in a fatal crash. This compares very favorably with a death risk per domestic flight of one in two million during the decade 1967–1976. Some believe that public concern about airline safety, in response to the impact of news stories, has played an important role in the dramatic improvement in safety in the airline industry.

The American public is aware that health care is less safe than some other environments, but to date, it has made few demands on the health care industry to demonstrate improvement. In a public opinion poll conducted by Louis Harris & Associates for the National Patient Safety Foundation, the health care environment was perceived as "moderately safe" (rated 4.9 on a scale of one through seven where one is not safe at all and seven is very safe).[109] Respondents viewed the health care environment as much safer than nuclear power or food handling, but somewhat less safe than airline travel or the work environment.

Americans have a very limited understanding of health care safety issues. When asked, What comes to mind when you think about patient safety issues in the health care environment? 28 percent of respondents did not mention anything, 20 percent mentioned exposure to infection, 13 percent cited the general level of care patients receive, and 11 percent cited qualifications of health professionals.[110] When asked about the main cause of medical mistakes, respondents most frequently cited carelessness or negligence (29 percent) of health care professionals, who are overworked, worried, or stressed (27 percent).

Most people learn about medical mistakes through anecdotes. More than four out of five respondents have heard about a situation in which a medical mistake was made.[111] When asked how they heard about the most recent medical mistake, 42 percent cited a friend or relative; 39 percent, television, newspaper, or radio; and 12 percent, personal experience.

Most people view medical mistakes as an "individual provider issue" rather than a failure in the process of delivering care in a complex delivery system. When asked about possible solutions to prevent medical mistakes, actions rated very effective by respondents were "keeping health care professionals with bad track records from providing care" (75 percent) and "better training of health care professionals" (69 percent).[112]

There are numerous factors that might contribute to the "disconnect" between public perceptions and actual health care error rates. The various accreditation and licensure programs for health care organizations and providers have been promoted as "Good Housekeeping Seals of Approval," yet they fail to provide adequate assurance of a safe environment. Reducing medical errors and improving patient safety are not an explicit focus of these processes. Even licensed and accredited organizations may have implemented only rudimentary systems and processes to ensure patient safety.

For the most part, media coverage has been limited to occasional reporting of anecdotal cases. The impact of anecdotal information on safety may also be less effective in health care than in the nuclear waste or airline industries, where an individual event often impacts dozens or hundreds of people at a time.

Patient safety is also hindered through the liability system and the threat of malpractice, which discourages the disclosure of errors. The discoverability of data under legal proceedings encourages silence about errors committed or observed. Most errors and safety issues go undetected and unreported, both externally and within health care organizations.

REFERENCES

1. Brennan, Troyen A.; Leape, Lucian L.; Laird, Nan M., et al. Incidence of adverse events and negligence in hospitalized patients: Results of the Harvard Medical Practice Study I. *N Engl J Med.* 324:370–376, 1991. See also: Leape, Lucian L.; Brennan, Troyen A.; Laird, Nan M., et al. The Nature of Adverse Events in Hospitalized Patients: Results of the Harvard Medical Practice Study II. *N Engl J Med.* 324(6):377–384, 1991. Thomas, Eric J.; Studdert, David M.; Burstin, Helen R., et al. Incidence and Types of Adverse Events and Negligent Care in Utah and Colorado. *Med Care* forthcoming Spring 2000.

2. Thomas, Eric J.; Studdert, David M.; Newhouse, Joseph P., et al. Costs of Medi-

cal Injuries in Utah and Colorado. *Inquiry.* 36:255–264, 1999. See also: Leape, et al., 1991. Brennan, et al., 1991.

3. American Hospital Association. Hospital Statistics. Chicago. 1999.

4. Centers for Disease Control and Prevention (National Center for Health Statistics). Deaths: Final Data for 1997. *National Vital Statistics Reports.* 47(19):27, 1999.

5. Centers for Disease Control and Prevention (National Center for Health Statistics). Births and Deaths: Preliminary Data for 1998. *National Vital Statistics Reports.* 47(25):6, 1999.

6. Thomas, et al., 1999.

7. Thomas, et al., 1999.

8. Thomas, et al., 1999.

9. Occupational Safety and Health Administration. The New OSHA: Reinventing Worker Safety and Health [Web Page]. Dec. 16, 1998. Available at: www.osha.gov/oshinfo/reinvent.html.

10. Bureau of Labor Statistics. National Census of Fatal Occupational Injuries, 1998. U.S. Department of Labor: Washington, D.C. August 1999.

11. Phillips, David P.; Christenfeld, Nicholas; Glynn, Laura M. Increase in US Medication-Error Deaths between 1983 and 1993. *Lancet.* 351:643–644, 1998.

12. Bates, David W.; Spell, Nathan; Cullen, David J., et al. The Costs of Adverse Drug Events in Hospitalized Patients. *JAMA.* 277:307–311, 1997.

13. National Wholesale Druggists' Association. *Industry Profile and Healthcare Factbook.* Reston, VA: 1998.

14. Hallas, Jesper; Haghfelt, Torben; Gram, Lars F., et al. Drug Related Admissions to a Cardiology Department: Frequency and Avoidability. *J Intern Med.* 228:379–384, 1990.

15. Willcox, Sharon M.; Himmelstein, David U.; Woolhandler, Steffie. Inappropriate Drug Prescribing for the Community Dwelling Elderly. *JAMA.* 272:292, 1994.

16. Knox, Richard. Prescription Errors Tied to Lack of Advice: Pharmacists Skirting Law, Massachusetts Study Finds. *Boston Globe.* February 10, 1999:(Metro);B1.

17. Einarson, Thomas R. Drug-Related Hospital Admissions. *Ann Pharmacother.* 27:832–840, 1993.

18. Reason, James T. Human Error. Cambridge, MA: Cambridge University Press; 1990.

19. Brennan, et al., 1991.

20. Leape, et al., 1991. See also Brennan, et al., 1991.

21. Leape, et al., 1991.

22. Manasse, Henri R. Jr. Medication Use in an Imperfect World: Drug Misadventuring as an Issue of Public Policy, part 1. *Am J Hosp Pharm.* 46:929–944, 1989.

23. Johnson, Jeffrey A., and Bootman, J. Lyle. Drug-Related Morbidity and Mortality: A Cost-of-Illness Model. *Arch Intern Med.* 155(18):1949–1956, 1995.

24. Victoroff, Michael S. The Right Intentions: Errors and Accountability. *J Fam Pract.* 45:38–39, 1997.

25. Andrews, Lori B.; Stocking, Carol; Krizek, Thomas, et al. An Alternative Strategy for Studying Adverse Events in Medical Care. *Lancet.* 349:309–313, 1997.

26. Vincent, Charles; Taylor-Adams, Sally and Stanhope, Nicole. Framework for Analysing Risk and Safety in Clinical Medicine. *BMJ.* 316(11):1154–1157, 1998.

27. Cook, Richard and Woods, David. Operating at the Sharp End: the Complexity

of Human Error. Bogner, Marilyn Sue, Ed. Human Errors in Medicine. Hillsdale, NJ: Lawrence Erlbaum Associates; 1994; pp. 255–310.

28. Nadzam, Deborah M. Development of Medication-Use Indicators by the Joint Commission on Accreditation of Health Care Organizations. *AJHP*. 48:1925–1930, 1991.

29. Brennan, et al., 1991.

30. Brennan, et al., 1991.

31. Leape, et al., 1991.

32. Brennan, et al., 1991.

33. Thomas, et al., 2000.

34. Thomas, et al., 1999.

35. Thomas, et al., 2000.

36. American Hospital Association. Hospital Statistics. Chicago. 1999. See also: Thomas, Eric J.; Studdert, David M.; Burstin, Helen R., et al. Incidence and Types of Adverse Events and Negligent Care in Utah and Colorado. *Med Care* forthcoming March 2000. See also: Thomas, Eric J.; Studdert, David M.; Newhouse, Joseph P., et al. Costs of Medical Injuries in Utah and Colorado. *Inquiry.* 36:255–264, 1999.

37. American Hospital Association. Hospital Statistics. Chicago. 1999. See also: Brennan, Troyen A.; Leape, Lucian L.; Laird, Nan M., et al. Incidence of adverse events and negligence in hospitalized patients: Results of the Harvard Medical Practice Study I. *N Engl J Med.* 324:370–376, 1991. See also: Leape, Lucian L.; Brennan, Troyen A.; Laird, Nan M., et al. The Nature of Adverse Events in Hospitalized Patients: Results of the Harvard Medical Practice Study II. *N Engl J Med.* 324(6):377–384, 1991.

38. Centers for Disease Control and Prevention (National Center for Health Statistics). Deaths: Final Data for 1997. *National Vital Statistics Reports* 47(19):27, 1999. See also: Centers for Disease Control and Prevention (National Center for Health Statistics). Births and Deaths: Preliminary Data for 1998. *National Vital Statistics Reports.* 47(25):6, 1999.

39. Andrews, et al., 1997.

40. Steel, Knight; Gertman, Paul M.; Crescenzi, Caroline, et al. Iatrogenic Illness on a General Medical Service at a University Hospital. *N Engl J Med.* 304:638–642, 1981.

41. Andrews, et al., 1997.

42. Dubois, Robert W. and Brook, Robert H. Preventable Deaths: Who, How Often, and Why? *Ann Intern Med.* 109:582–589, 1988.

43. Bedell, Susanne E.; Deitz, David C.; Leeman, David, et al. Incidence and Characteristics of Preventable Iatrogenic Cardiac Arrests. *JAMA.* 265(21):2815–2820, 1995.

44. McGuire, Hunter H.; Horsley, J. Shelton; Salter, David R., et al. Measuring and Managing Quality of Surgery: Statistical vs Incidental Approaches. *Arch Surg.* 127:733–737, 1992.

45. Cooper, Jeffrey B.; Newbower, Ronald S.; Long, Charlene D., et al. Preventable Anesthesia Mishaps: A Study of Human Factors. *Anesthesiology.* 49:399–406, 1978.

46. Gaba, David M. Human Error in Anesthetic Mishaps. *Int Anesthesiol Clin.* 27(3):137–147, 1989.

47. Duncan, Peter G., and Cohen, Marsha M. Postoperative Complications: Factors of Significance to Anaesthetic Practice. *Can J Anaesth.* 34:2–8, 1987.

48. Cohen, Marsha M.; Duncan, Peter G.; Pope, William D. B., et al. A Survey of 112,000 Anaesthetics at One Teaching Hospital (1975–1983). *Can Anaesth Soc J.* 33:22–31, 1986.

49. Sentinel Events: Approaches to Error Reduction and Prevention. *Jt Comm J Qual Improv*. 24(4):175–186, 1998.

50. Chassin, Mark R. Is Health Care Ready for Six Sigma Quality? *Milbank Q.* 764:565–591, 1998.

51. Bhasale, Alice L.; Miller, Graeme C.; Reid, Sharon E., et al. Analysing Potential Harm in Australian General Practice: an Incident-Monitoring Study. *MJA*. 169:73–76, 1998.

52. National Wholesale Druggists' Association. *Industry Profile and Healthcare Factbook, op cit.*

53. Manasse, 1989.

54. Phillips, et al., 1998.

55. Bates, David W.; Boyle, Deborah L.; Vander Vilet, Martha, et al. Relationship between Medication Errors and Adverse Drug Events. *J Gen Intern Med*. 10:199–205, 1995.

56. Lesar, Timothy S.; Briceland, Laurie, and Stein, Daniel S. Factors Related to Errors in Medication Prescribing. *JAMA*. 277(4):312–317, 1997.

57. Bates, David W.; Cullen, David J.; Laird, Nan M., et al. Incidence of Adverse Drug Events and Potential Adverse Drug Events: Implications for Prevention. *JAMA*. 274:29–34, 1995.

58. Bates, David W.; Leape, Lucian L., and Petrycki, Stanley. Incidence and Preventability of Adverse Drug Events in Hospitalized Adults. *J Gen Intern Med*. 8:289–294, 1993.

59. Lesar, Briceland, and Stein, 1997.

60. Koren, Gideon and Haslam, Robert H. Pediatric Medication Errors: Predicting and Preventing Tenfold Disasters. *J Clin Pharmacol*. 34:1043–1045, 1994.

61. Perlstein, Paul H.; Callison, Cornelia; White, Mary, et al. Errors in Drug Computations During Newborn Intensive Care. *Am J Dis Child*. 33:376–379, 1979.

62. Folli, Hugo L.; Poole, Robert L.; Benitz, William E., et al. Medication Error Prevention by Clinical Pharmacists in Two Children's Hospitals. *Pediatrics*. 79:718–722, 1987.

63. Raju, Tonse N. K.; Kecskes, Susan; Thornton, John P., et al. Medication Errors in Neonatal and Paediatric Intensive-Care Units. *Lancet*. 374–376, 1989.

64. Cullen, David J.; Sweitzer, Bobbie Jean; Bates, David W., et al. Preventable Adverse Drug Events in Hospitalized Patients: A Comparative Study of Intensive Care and General Care Units. *Crit Care Med*. 25(8):1289–1297, 1997.

65. Manasse, 1989.

66. Davies, D.M., ed. Textbook on Adverse Drug Reactions, 3rd. ed. Oxford: Oxford University Press; 1985.

67. Griffin, J. P., and Weber, J. C. P. Voluntary Systems of Adverse Reaction Reporting—Part I. *Adverse Drug React Acute Poisoning Rev*. 4:213–230, 1985.

68. Griffin, J. P., and Weber, J. C. P. Voluntary Systems of Adverse Reaction Reporting—Part II. *Adverse Drug React Acute Poisoning Rev*. 5:23–25, 1986.

69. Cullen, David J.; Bates, David W.; Small, Stephen D., et al. The Incident Reporting System Does Not Detect Adverse Drug Events. *Jt Comm J Qual Improv*. 21(10):541–548, 1995.

70. Classen, David C.; Pestonik, Stanley, L.; Evans, Scott; Burke, John P., et al. Com-

puterized Surveillance of Adverse Drug Events in Hospital Patients. *JAMA.* 266(20):2847–2851.

71. Beard, Keith. Adverse Reactions as a Cause of Hospital Admissions in the Aged. *Drug Aging.* 2:356–361, 1992.

72. Roughead, Elizabeth E.; Gilbert, Andrew L.; Primrose, J. G., et al. Drug-Related Hospital Admissions: A Review of Australian Studies Published 1998–1996. *Med J. Aust.* 168:405–408, 1998.

73. Burnum, John F. Preventability of Adverse Drug Reactions. *Ann Intern Med.* 85:80, 1976.

74. Schneitman-McIntire, Orinda.; Farnen, Tracy A.; Gordon, Nancy, et al. Medication Misadventures Resulting in Emergency Department Visits at an HMO Medical Center. *Am J Health Syst Pharm.* 3:1416–1422, 1996.

75. Sullivan, Sean D.; Kreling, David H.; Hazlet, Thomas K., et al. Noncompliance with Medication Regimens and Subsequent Hospitalizations: A Literature Analysis and Cost of Hospitalization Estimate. *J Res Pharm Econom.* 2(2):19–33, 1990.

76. Einarson, 1993.

77. Thomas, et al., 2000.

78. Dubois, Robert W. and Brook, Robert H. Preventable Deaths: Who, How Often, and Why? *Ann Int Med.* 109:582–589, 1988.

79. Bedell, Susanna E.; Deitz, David C.; Leeman, David; Delbanco, Thomas, L. Incidence and Characteristics of Preventable Iatrogenic Cardiac Arrests. *JAMA.* 265:2815–2820, 1991.

80. Lesar, Briceland, and Stein, 1997.

81. Willcox, Sharon M.; Himmelstein, David U.; Woolhandler, Steffie, et al. Inappropriate Drug Prescribing for the Community Dwelling Elderly, *op cit.*

82. Hallas, et al., 1997.

83. Wilson, Dirk G.; McArtney, R. G.; Newcombe, Robert G., et al. Medication Errors in Paediatric Practice: Insights from a Continuous Quality Improvement Approach. *Eur J Pediatr.* 157:769–774, 1998.

84. Burnum, 1976.

85. Beers, Mark H.; Storrie, Michele; and Lee, Genell. Potential Adverse Drug Interactions in the Emergency Room. *Ann Intern Med.* 112:61–64, 1990.

86. Knox, 1999.

87. Bates, et al., 1995.

88. Davis, Neil M. and Cohen, Michael R. Medication Errors: Causes and Prevention. Philadelphia: George F. Stickley Co., 1981.

89. Folli, et al., 1987.

90. Greenberg, Jay; Leutz, Walter; Greenlick, Merwyn, et al. The Social HMO Demonstration: Early Experience. *Health Affairs.* 7:66, 1988.

91. Strandberg, Lee R. Drugs as a Reason for Nursing Home Admissions. *Am Health Care Assoc J.* 10:20–23, 1984.

92. Leape, Lucian L.; Bates, David W., and Cullen, David J. Systems Analysis of Adverse Drug Events. *JAMA.* 274:35–43, 1995.

93. Bates, et al., 1995.

94. Folli, et al., 1987.

95. Blum, Keith V.; Abel, S.R.; Urbanski, Chris J., et al. Medication Error Prevention by Pharmacists. *Am J Hosp Pharm.* 45:1902–1903, 1988

96. Thomas, et al., 1999.

97. Alliance for Aging Research. When Medicine Hurts Instead of Helps. Washington, DC: The Alliance for Aging Research; 1998.

98. Johnson, et al., 1995.

99. Hallas, et al., 1997.

100. Willcox, et al., 1994.

101. Knox, 1999.

102. Einarson, 1993.

103. Bates, David W., et al. The Costs of Adverse Drug Events in Hospitalized Patients, *op cit*, 1995.

104. Classen, David C.; Pestotnik, Stanley L.; Evans, R. Scott, et al. Adverse Drug Events in Hospitalized Patients: Excess Length of Stay, Extra Costs, and Attributable Mortality. *JAMA*. 277:301–306, 1997.

105. Schneider, Philip J.; Gift, Maja G.; Lee, Yu-Ping, et al. Cost of Medication-Related Problems at a University Hospital. *Am J Health Syst Pharm*. 52:2415–2418, 1995.

106. Bloom, Bernard S. Cost of Treating Arthritis and NSAID-Related Gastrointestinal Side-Effects. *Aliment Pharmacol Ther*. 1(Suppl 2):131–138, 1998.

107. Bootman, J. Lyle; Harrison, LTC Donald L., and Cox, Emily. The Health Care Cost of Drug-Related Morbidity and Mortality in Nursing Facilities. *Arch Intern Med*. 157(18):2089–2096, 1997.

108. Federal Aviation Administration, Office of System Safety. Aviation Safety Reporting System (ASRS) Database [Web Page]. 1999. Available at: http://nasdac.faa.gov/safety data.

109. National Patient Safety Foundation. Diverse Groups Come Together to Improve Health Care Safety Through the National Patient Safety Foundation [Web Page]. 1997 Aug 29. Available at: http://www.ama-assn.org/med-sci/npsf/pr897.htm. Note: press release.

110. National Patient Safety Foundation, 1997.

111. National Patient Safety Foundation, 1997.

112. National Patient Safety Foundation, 1997.

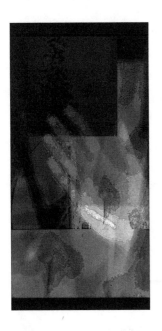

3
Why Do
Errors Happen?

The common initial reaction when an error occurs is to find and blame someone. However, even apparently single events or errors are due most often to the convergence of multiple contributing factors. Blaming an individual does not change these factors and the same error is likely to recur. Preventing errors and improving safety for patients require a systems approach in order to modify the conditions that contribute to errors. People working in health care are among the most educated and dedicated workforce in any industry. The problem is not bad people; the problem is that the system needs to be made safer.

This chapter covers two key areas. First, definitions of several key terms are offered. This is important because there is no agreed-upon terminology for talking about this issue.[1] Second, the emphasis in this chapter (and in this report generally) is about how to make systems safer; its primary focus is not on "getting rid of bad apples," or individuals with patterns of poor performance. The underlying assumption is that lasting and broad-based safety improvements in an industry can be brought about through a systems approach.

Finally, it should be noted that although the examples may draw more from inpatient or institutional settings, errors occur in all settings. The concepts presented in this chapter are just as applicable to ambulatory care, home care, community pharmacies, or any other setting in which health care is delivered.

This chapter uses a case study to illustrate a series of definitions and concepts in patient safety. After presentation of the case study, the chapter will define what comprises a system, how accidents occur, how human error contributes to accidents and how these elements fit into a broader concept of safety. The case study will be referenced to illustrate several of the concepts. The next section will examine whether certain types of systems are more prone to accidents than others. Finally, after a short discussion of the study of human factors, the chapter summarizes what health care can learn from other industries about safety.

An Illustrative Case in Patient Safety

Infusion devices are mechanical devices that administer intravenous solutions containing drugs to patients. A patient was undergoing a cardiac procedure. This patient had a tendency toward being hypertensive and this was known to the staff.

As part of the routine set-up for surgery, a nurse assembled three different infusion devices. The nurse was a new member of the team in the operating room; she had just started working at the hospital a few weeks before. The other members of the team had been working together for at least six months. The nurse was being very careful when setting up the devices because one of them was a slightly different model than she had used before.

Each infusion device administered a different medication that would be used during surgery. For each medication, the infusion device had to be programmed according to how much medication would flow into the patient (calculated as "cc's/hour"). The medications had different concentrations and each required calculation of the correct dose for that specific patient. The correct cc's/hour were programmed into the infusion devices.

The anesthesiologist, who monitors and uses the infusion devices during surgery, usually arrived for surgery while the nurse was completing her set-up of the infusion devices and was able to check them over. This particular morning, the anesthesiologist was running behind from a previous surgery. When he arrived in the operating room, the rest of the team was ready to start. The anesthesiologist quickly glanced at the set-up and accepted the report as given to him by the nurse.

One of the infusion devices was started at the beginning of surgery. About

WHY DO ACCIDENTS HAPPEN?

Major accidents, such as Three Mile Island or the *Challenger* accident, grab people's attention and make the front page of newspapers. Because they usually affect only one individual at a time, accidents in health care delivery are less visible and dramatic than those in other industries. Except for celebrated cases, such as Betsy Lehman (the *Boston Globe* reporter who died from an overdose during chemotherapy) or Willie King (who had the wrong leg amputated),[2] they are rarely noticed. However, accidents are a form of information about a system.[3] They represent places in which the system failed and the breakdown resulted in harm.

The ideas in this section rely heavily upon the work of Charles Perrow

---

halfway through the surgery, the patient's blood pressure began to rise. The anesthesiologist tried to counteract this by starting one of the other infusion devices that had been set up earlier. He checked the drip chamber in the intravenous (IV) tubing and did not see any drips. He checked the IV tubing and found a closed clamp, which he opened. At this point, the second device signaled an occlusion, or blockage, in the tubing by sounding an alarm and flashing an error message. The anesthesiologist found a closed clamp in this tubing as well, opened it, pressed the re-start button and the device resumed pumping without further difficulty. He returned to the first device that he had started and found that there had been a free flow of fluid and medication to the patient, resulting in an overdose. The team responded appropriately and the patient recovered without further incident.

The case was reviewed two weeks later at the hospital's "morbidity and mortality" committee meeting, where the hospital staff reviews cases that encountered a problem to identify what happened and how to avoid a recurrence. The IV tubing had been removed from the device and discarded. The bioengineering service had checked the pump and found it to be functioning accurately. It was not possible to determine whether the tubing had been inserted incorrectly into the device, whether the infusion rate had been set incorrectly or changed while the device was in use, or whether the device had malfunctioned unexpectedly. The anesthesiologist was convinced that the tubing had been inserted incorrectly, so that when the clamp was open the fluid was able to flow freely rather than being controlled by the infusion device. The nurse felt the anesthesiologist had failed to check the infusion system adequately before turning on the devices. Neither knew whether it was possible for an infusion device to have a safety mechansim built into it that would prevent free flows from happening.

and James Reason, among others. Charles Perrow's analysis of the accident at Three Mile Island identified how systems can cause or prevent accidents.[4] James Reason extended the thinking by analyzing multiple accidents to examine the role of systems and the human contribution to accidents.[5] *"A system is a set of interdependent elements interacting to achieve a common aim. The elements may be both human and non-human (equipment, technologies, etc.)."*

Systems can be very large and far-reaching, or they can be more localized. In health care, a system can be an integrated delivery system, a centrally owned multihospital system, or a virtual system comprised of many different partners over a wide geographic area. However, an operating room or an obstetrical unit is also a type of system. Furthermore, any element in a system probably belongs to multiple systems. For example, one operating room is part of a surgical department, which is part of a hospital, which is part of a larger health care delivery system. The variable size, scope, and membership of systems make them difficult to analyze and understand.

In the case study, one of the systems used during surgery is the automated, medication adminstration system, which includes the equipment, the people, their interactions with each other and with the equipment, the procedures in place, and the physical design of the surgical suite in which the equipment and people function.

When large systems fail, it is due to multiple faults that occur together in an unanticipated interaction,[6] creating a chain of events in which the faults grow and evolve.[7] Their accumulation results in an accident. *"An accident is an event that involves damage to a defined system that disrupts the ongoing or future output of that system."*[8]

The *Challenger* failed because of a combination of brittle O-ring seals, unexpected cold weather, reliance on the seals in the design of the boosters, and change in the roles of the contractor and NASA. Individually, no one factor caused the event, but when they came together, disaster struck. Perrow uses a DEPOSE (**D**esign, **E**quipment **P**rocedures, **O**perators, **S**upplies and materials, and **E**nvironment) framework to identify the potential sources of failures. In evaluating the environment, some researchers explicitly include organizational design and characteristics.[9]

In the case study, the accident was a breakdown in the delivery of IV medications during surgery.

The complex coincidences that cause systems to fail could rarely have been foreseen by the people involved. As a result, they are reviewed only in hindsight; however, knowing the outcome of an event influences how we assess past events.[10] *Hindsight bias* means that things that were not seen or understood at the time of the accident seem obvious in retrospect. Hindsight bias also misleads a reviewer into simplifying the causes of an accident, highlighting a single element as the cause and overlooking multiple contributing factors. Given that the information about an accident is spread over many participants, none of whom may have complete information,[11] hindsight bias makes it easy to arrive at a simple solution or to blame an individual, but difficult to determine what really went wrong.

Although many features of systems and accidents in other industries are also found in health care, there are important differences. In most other industries, when an accident occurs the worker and the company are directly affected. There is a saying that the pilot is always the first at the scene of an airline accident. In health care, the damage happens to a third party; the patient is harmed; the health professional or the organization, only rarely. Furthermore, harm occurs to only one patient at a time; not whole groups of patients, making the accident less visible. *

In any industry, one of the greatest contributors to accidents is human error. Perrow has estimated that, on average, 60–80 percent of accidents involve human error. There is reason to believe that this is equally true in health. An analysis of anesthesia found that human error was involved in 82 percent of preventable incidents; the remainder involved mainly equipment failure.[12] Even when equipment failure occurs, it can be exacerbated by human error.[13] However, saying that an accident is due to human error is not the same as assigning blame. Humans commit errors for a variety of

---

*Public health has made an effort to eliminate the term, "accident," replacing it with unintentional injuries, consistent with the nomenclature of the International Classification of Diseases. However, this report is not focused specifically on injury since an accident may or may not result in injury. See Institute of Medicine, *Reducing the Burden of Injury*, eds. Richard J. Bonnie, Carolyn Fulco and Catharyn Liverman. Washington, D.C., National Academy Press, 1999).

expected and unexpected reasons, which are discussed in more detail in the next two sections.

Understanding Errors

The work of Reason provides a good understanding of errors. He defines an error as the failure of a planned sequence of mental or physical activities to achieve its intended outcome when these failures cannot be attributed to chance.[14] It is important to note the inclusion of "intention." According to Reason, error is not meaningful without the consideration of intention. That is, it has no meaning when applied to unintentional behaviors because errors depend on two kinds of failure, either actions do not go as intended or the intended action is not the correct one. In the first case, the desired outcome may or may not be achieved; in the second case, the desired outcome cannot be achieved.

Reason differentiates between slips or lapses and mistakes. A slip or lapse occurs when the action conducted is not what was intended. It is an error of execution. The difference between a slip and a lapse is that a slip is observable and a lapse is not. For example, turning the wrong knob on a piece of equipment would be a slip; not being able to recall something from memory is a lapse.

In a mistake, the action proceeds as planned but fails to achieve its intended outcome because the planned action was wrong. The situation might have been assessed incorrectly, and/or there could have been a lack of knowledge of the situation. In a mistake, the original intention is inadequate; a failure of planning is involved.

In medicine, slips, lapses, and mistakes are all serious and can potentially harm patients. For example, in medicine, a slip might be involved if the physician chooses an appropriate medication, writes 10 mg when the intention was to write 1 mg. The original intention is correct (the correct medication was chosen given the patient's condition), but the action did not proceed as planned. On the other hand, a mistake in medicine might involve selecting the wrong drug because the diagnosis is wrong. In this case, the situation was misassessed and the action planned is wrong. If the terms "slip" and "mistake" are used, it is important not to equate slip with "minor." Patients can die from slips as well as mistakes.

For this report, *error is defined as the failure of a planned action to be completed as intended (e.g., error of execution) or the use of a wrong plan to achieve an aim (e.g., error of planning)*. From the patient's perspective, not only should a medical intervention proceed properly and safely, it should be the correct intervention for the particular condition. This report addresses primarily the first concern, errors of execution, since they have their own epidemiology, causes, and remedies that are different from errors in planning. Subsequent reports from the Quality of Health Care in America project will consider the full range of quality-related issues, sometimes classified as overuse, underuse and misuse.[15]

Latent and Active Errors

In considering how humans contribute to error, it is important to distinguish between active and latent errors.[16] *Active errors occur at the level of the frontline operator, and their effects are felt almost immediately.* This is sometimes called the sharp end.[17] *Latent errors tend to be removed from the direct control of the operator and include things such as poor design, incorrect installation, faulty maintenance, bad management decisions, and poorly structured organizations.* These are called the blunt end. The active error is that the pilot crashed the plane. The latent error is that a previously undiscovered design malfunction caused the plane to roll unexpectedly in a way the pilot could not control and the plane crashed.

In the case study, the active error was the free flow of the medication from the infusion device.

Latent errors pose the greatest threat to safety in a complex system because they are often unrecognized and have the capacity to result in multiple types of active errors. Analysis of the *Challenger* accident traced contributing events back nine years. In the Three Mile Island accident, latent errors were traced back two years.[18] Latent errors can be difficult for the people working in the system to notice since the errors may be hidden in the design of routine processes in computer programs or in the structure or management of the organization. People also become accustomed to design defects and learn to work around them, so they are often not recognized.

In her book about the *Challenger* explosion, Vaughan describes the "normalization of deviance" in which small changes in behavior became the norm and expanded the boundaries so that additional deviations became acceptable.[19] When deviant events become acceptable, the potential for errors is created because signals are overlooked or misinterpreted and accumulate without being noticed.

Current responses to errors tend to focus on the active errors by punishing individuals (e.g., firing or suing them), retraining or other responses aimed at preventing recurrence of the active error. Although a punitive response may be appropriate in some cases (e.g., deliberate malfeasance), it is not an effective way to prevent recurrence. Because large system failures represent latent failures coming together in unexpected ways, they appear to be unique in retrospect. Since the same mix of factors is unlikely to occur again, efforts to prevent specific active errors are not likely to make the system any safer.[20]

In our case study, a number of latent failures were present:

- Multiple infusion devices were used in parallel during this cardiac surgery. Three devices were set up, each requiring many steps. each step in the assembly presents a possibility for failure that could disrupt the entire system.
- Each of the three different medications had to be programmed into the infusion device with the correct dose for that patient.
- Possible scheduling problems in the operating suites may have contributed to the anesthesiologist having insufficient time to check the devices before surgery.
- A new nurse on the team may have interrupted the "normal" flow between the team members, especially communication between the anesthesiologist and the nurse setting up the devices. There was no standardized list of checks between the nurse and anesthesiologist before starting the procedure.
- Training of new team members may be insufficient since the nurse found herself assembling a device that was a slightly different model. As a new employee, she may have been hesitant to ask for help or may not have known who to ask.

Focusing on active errors lets the latent failures remain in the system, and their accumulation actually makes the system more prone to future failure.[21] Discovering and fixing latent failures, and decreasing their duration, are likely to have a greater effect on building safer systems than efforts to minimize active errors at the point at which they occur.

In the case study, a typical response would have been to retrain the nurse on how to assemble the equipment properly. However, this would have had no effect on weaknesses in equipment design, team management and communications, scheduling problems, or orienting new staff. Thus, free flow errors would likely recur.

Understanding Safety

Most of this chapter thus far has drawn on Perrow's normal accident theory, which believes that accident are inevitable in certain systems. Although they may be rare, accidents are "normal" in complex, high technology industries. In contrast to studying the causes of accident and errors, other researchers have focused on the characteristics that make certain industries, such as military aircraft carriers or chemical processing, highly reliable.[22] High reliability theory believes that accidents can be prevented through good organizational design and management.[23] Characteristics of highly reliable industries include an organizational commitment to safety, high levels of redundancy in personnel and safety measures, and a strong organizational culture for continuous learning and willingness to change.[24] Correct performance and error can be viewed as "two sides of the same coin."[25] Although accidents may occur, systems can be designed to be safer so that accidents are very rare.

The National Patient Safety Foundation has defined patient safety as the avoidance, prevention and amelioration of adverse outcomes or injuries stemming from the processes of health care.[26] Safety does not reside in a person, device or department, but emerges from the interactions of components of a system. Others have specifically examined pharmaceutical safety and defined it to include maximizing therapeutic benefit, reducing risk, and eliminating harm.[27] That is, benefit relates to risk. Other experts have also defined safety as a relative concept. Brewer and Colditz suggest that the acceptability of an adverse event depends on the seriousness of the underlying illness and the availability of alternative treatments.[28] The committee's focus, however, was not on the patient's response to a treatment, but rather on the ability of a system to deliver care safely. From this perspective, the committee believes that there is a level of safety that can and should be ensured. Safety is relative only in that it continues to evolve over time and, when risks do become known, they become part of the safety requirements.

Safety is more than just the absence of errors. Safety has multiple dimensions, including the following:

- an outlook that recognizes that health care is complex and risky and that solutions are found in the broader systems context;
- a set of processes that identify, evaluate, and minimize hazards and are continuously improving, and
- an outcome that is manifested by fewer medical errors and minimized risk or hazard.[29]

For this report, *safety is defined as freedom from accidental injury*. This simple definition recognizes that from the patient's perspective, the primary safety goal is to prevent accidental injuries. If an environment is safe, the risk of accidents is lower. Making environments safer means looking at processes of care to reduce defects in the process or departures from the way things should have been done. Ensuring patient safety, therefore, involves the establishment of operational systems and processes that increase the reliability of patient care.

ARE SOME TYPES OF SYSTEMS MORE PRONE TO ACCIDENTS?

Accidents are more likely to happen in certain types of systems. When they do occur, they represent failures in the way systems are designed. The primary objective of systems design ought to be to make it difficult for accidents and errors to occur and to minimize damage if they do occur.[30]

Perrow characterizes systems according to two important dimensions: complexity and tight or loose coupling.[31] Systems that are more complex and tightly coupled are more prone to accidents and have to be made more reliable.[32] In Reason's words, complex and tightly coupled systems can "spring nasty surprises."[33]

In complex systems, one component of the system can interact with multiple other components, sometimes in unexpected or invisible ways. Although all systems have many parts that interact, the problem arises when one part serves multiple functions because if this part fails, all of the dependent functions fail as well. Complex systems are characterized by specialization and interdependency. Complex systems also tend to have multiple feedback loops, and to receive information indirectly, and because of specialization, there is little chance of substituting or reassigning personnel or other resources.

In contrast to complex systems, linear systems contain interactions that are expected in the usual and familiar production sequence. One component of the system interacts with the component immediately preceding it in the production process and the component following it. Linear systems tend to have segregated subsystems, few feedback loops, and easy substitutions (less specialization).

An example of complexity is the concern with year 2000 (Y2K) computer problems. A failure in one part of the system can unexpectedly interrupt other parts, and all of the interrelated processes that can be affected are not yet visible. Complexity is also the reason that changes in long-standing production processes must be made cautiously.[34] When tasks are distributed across a team, for example, many interactions that are critical to the process may not be noticed until they are changed or removed.

Coupling is a mechanical term meaning that there is no slack or buffer between two items. Large systems that are tightly coupled have more time-dependent processes and sequences that are more fixed (e.g., y depends on x having been done). There is often only one way to reach a goal. Compared to tightly coupled systems, loosely coupled systems can tolerate processing delays, can reorder the sequence of production, and can employ alternative methods or resources.

All systems have linear interactions; however, some systems additionally experience greater complexity. Complex interactions contribute to accidents because they can confuse operators. Tight coupling contributes to accidents because things unravel too quickly and prevent errors from being intercepted or prevent speedy recovery from an event.[35] Because of complexity and coupling, small failures can grow into large accidents.

In the case study, the medication adminstration system was both complex and tightly coupled. The complexity arises from three devices functioning simultaneously, in close proximity, and two having problems at the same time. The tight coupling arises from the steps involved in making the system work properly, from the steps required to assemble three devices, to the calculation of correct medication dosage levels, to the operation of multiple devices during surgery, to the responses when alarms start going off.

Although there are not firm assignments, Perrow considered nuclear power plants, nuclear weapons handling, and aircraft to be complex, tightly coupled systems.[36] Multiple processes are happening simultaneously, and failure in one area can interrupt another. Dams and rail transportation are considered tightly coupled because the steps in production are closely linked, but linear because there are few unexpected interactions. Universities are considered complex, but loosely coupled, since the impact of a decision in one area can likely be limited to that area.

Perrow did not classify health care as a system, but others have suggested that health care is complex and tightly coupled.[37] The activities in the typical emergency room, surgical suite, or intensive care unit exemplify complex and tightly coupled systems. Therefore, the delivery of health care services may be classified as an industry prone to accidents.[38]

Complex, tightly coupled systems have to be made more reliable.[39] One of the advantages of having systems is that it is possible to build in more defenses against failure. Systems that are more complex, tightly coupled, and are more prone to accidents can reduce the likelihood of accidents by simplifying and standardizing processes, building in redundancy, developing backup systems, and so forth.

Another aspect of making systems more reliable has to do with organizational design and team performance. Since these are part of activities within organizations, they are discussed in Chapter 8.

Conditions That Create Errors

Factors can intervene between the design of a system and the production process that creates conditions in which errors are more likely to happen. James Reason refers to these factors as psychological precursors or preconditions.[40] Although good managerial decisions are required for safe and efficient production, they are not sufficient. There is also a need to have the right equipment, well-maintained and reliable; a skilled and knowledgeable workforce; reasonable work schedules, well-designed jobs; clear guidance on desired and undesired performance, et cetera. Factors such as these are the precursors or preconditions for safe production processes.

Any given precondition can contribute to a large number of unsafe acts. For example, training deficiencies can show up as high workload, undue time pressure, inappropriate perception of hazards, or motivational difficulties.[41] Preconditions are latent failures embedded in the system. Designing safe systems means taking into account people's psychological limits and either seeking ways to eliminate the preconditions or intervening to minimize their consequences. Job design, equipment selection and use, operational procedures, work schedules, and so forth, are all factors in the production process that can be designed for safety.

One specific type of precondition that receives a lot of attention is technology. The occurrence of human error creates the perception that humans are unreliable and inefficient. One response to this has been to find the unreliable person who committed the error and focus on preventing him or her from doing it again. Another response has been to increase the use of technology to automate processes so as to remove opportunities for humans to make errors. The growth of technology over the past several decades has contributed to system complexity so this particular issue is highlighted here.

Technology changes the tasks that people do by shifting the workload and eliminating human decision making.[42] Where a worker previously may have overseen an entire production process, he or she may intervene now only in the last few steps if the previous steps are automated. For example, flying an aircraft has become more automated, which has helped reduce workload during nonpeak periods. During peak times, such as take-off and landing, there may be more processes to monitor and information to interpret.

Furthermore, the operator must still do things that cannot be automated. This usually involves having to monitor automated systems for rare, abnormal events[43] because machines cannot deal with infrequent events in a constantly changing environment.[44] Fortunately, automated systems rarely fail. Unfortunately, this means that operators do not practice basic skills, so workers lose skills in exactly the activities they need in order to take over when something goes wrong.

Automation makes systems more "opaque" to people who manage, maintain, and operate them.[45] Processes that are automated are less visible because machines intervene between the person and the task. For example, automation means that people have less hands-on contact with processes and are elevated to more supervisory and planning tasks. Direct information is filtered through a machine (e.g., a computer), and operators run the risk of having too much information to interpret or of not getting the right information.

In the case study, the infusion device administered the medication and the professional monitored the process, intervening when problems arose. The medication administration process was "opaque" in that the device provided no feedback to the user when the medication flowed freely and minimal feedback when the medication flow was blocked.

One of the advantages of technology is that it can enhance human performance to the extent that the human plus technology is more powerful than either is alone.[46] Good machines can question the actions of operators, offer advice, and examine a range of alternative possibilities that humans cannot possibly remember. In medicine, automated order entry systems or decision support systems have this aim. However, technology can also create new demands on operators. For example, a new piece of equipment may provide more precise measurements, but also demand better precision from the operator for the equipment to work properly.[47] Devices that have not been standardized, or that work and look differently, increase the likelihood of operator errors. Equipment may not be designed using human factors principles to account for the human–machine interface.[48]

In the case study, safer systems could have been designed by taking into consideration characteristics of how people use machines and interact with each other in teams. For example:

- Redesign the devices to default to a safe mode
- Reduce the difficulties of using multiple devices simultaneously
- Minimize the variety of equipment models purchased
- Implement clear procedures for checking equipment, supplies, etc., prior to begixnning surgery
- Orient and train new staff with the team(s) with which they will work
- Provide a supportive environment for identifying and communicating about errors for organizational learning and change to prevent errors.

Technology also has to be recognized as a "member" of the work team. When technology shifts workloads, it also shifts the interactions between team members. Where processes may have been monitored by several people, technology can permit the task to be accomplished by fewer people. This affects the distributed nature of the job in which tasks are shared among several people and may influence the ability to discover and recover from errors.[49]

In this context, technology does not involve just computers and information technology. It includes "techniques, drugs, equipment and procedures used by health care professionals in delivering medical care to individuals and the systems within which such care is delivered."[50] Additionally, the use of the term technology is not restricted to the technology employed by health care professionals. It can also include people at home of different ages, visual abilities, languages, and so forth, who must use different kinds of medical equipment and devices. As more care shifts to ambulatory and home settings, the use of medical technology by non-health professionals can be expected to take on increasing importance.

RESEARCH ON HUMAN FACTORS

Research in the area of human factors is just beginning to be applied to health care. It borrows from the disciplines of industrial engineering and psychology. *Human factors is defined as the study of the interrelationships between humans, the tools they use, and the environment in which they live and work.*[51]

In the context of this report, a human factors approach is used to understand where and why systems or processes break down. This approach examines the process of error, looking at the causes, circumstances, conditions, associated procedures and devices and other factors connected with the event. Studying human performance can result in the creation of safer systems and the reduction of conditions that lead to errors. However, not all errors are related to human factors. Although equipment and materials should take into account the design of the way people use them, human factors may not resolve instances of equipment breakdown or material failure.

Much of the work in human factors is on improving the human–system interface by designing better systems and processes.[52] This might include, for example, simplifying and standardizing procedures, building in redundancy to provide backup and opportunities for recovery, improving communications and coordination within teams, or redesigning equipment to improve the human–machine interface.

Two approaches have typically been used in human factors analysis. The first is critical incident analysis. Critical incident analysis examines a significant or pivotal occurrence to understand where the system broke down, why the incident occurred, and the circumstances surrounding the incident.[53] Analyzing critical incidents, whether or not the event actually leads to a bad outcome, provides an understanding of the conditions that produced an actual error or the risk of error and contributing factors.

In the case study, researchers with expertise in human factors could have helped the team investigate the problem. They could examine how the device performed under different circumstances (e.g., what the alarms and displays did when the medication flow changed), varying the setup and operation of the infusion device to observe how it performed under normal and abnormal conditions. They could observe how the staff used the particular infusion device during surgery and how they interacted with the use of multiple infusion devices.

A critical incident analysis in anesthesia found that human error was involved in 82 percent of preventable incidents. The study identified the most frequent categories of error and the riskiest steps in the process of administering anesthesia. Recommended corrective actions included such things as labeling and packaging strategies to highlight differences among anesthesiologists in the way they prepared their workspace, training issues for residents, work–rest cycles, how relief and replacement processes could be improved, and equipment improvements (e.g., standardizing equipment in terms of the shape of knobs and the direction in which they turn).

Another analytic approach is referred to as "naturalistic decision making."[54] This approach examines the way people make decisions in their natural work settings. It considers all of the factors that are typically controlled for in a laboratory-type evaluation, such as time pressure, noise and other distractions, insufficient information, and competing goals. In this method, the researcher goes out with workers in various fields, such as firefighters or nurses, observes them in practice, and then walks them through to reconstruct various incidents. The analysis uncovers the factors weighed and the processes used in making decisions when faced with ambiguous information under time pressure.

In terms of applying human factors research, David Woods of Ohio State University describes a process of reporting, investigation, innovation, and dissemination (David Woods, personal communication, December 17, 1998). Reporting or other means of identifying errors tells people where errors are occurring and where improvements can be made. The investigation stage uses human factors and other analyses to determine the contributing factors and circumstances that created the conditions in which errors could occur. The design of safer systems provides opportunities for innovation and working with early adopters to test out new approaches. Finally, dissemination of innovation throughout the industry shifts the baseline for performance. The experience of the early adopters redefines what is possible and provides models for implementation.

Aviation has long analyzed the role of human factors in performance. The Ames Research Center (part of the National Aeronautics and Space Administration) has examined areas related to information technology, automation, and the use of simulators for training in basic and crisis skills, for example. Other recent projects include detecting and correcting errors in flight; interruptions, distractions and lapses of attention in the cockpit; and designing information displays to assist pilots in maintaining awareness of their situation during flight.[55]

SUMMARY

The following key points can be summarized from this chapter.

1. Some systems are more prone to accidents than others because of the way the components are tied together. Health care services is a complex and technological industry prone to accidents.

2. Much can be done to make systems more reliable and safe. When large systems fail, it is due to multiple faults that occur together.

3. One of the greatest contributors to accidents in any industry including health care, is human error. However, saying that an accident is due to human error is not the same as assigning blame because most human errors are induced by system failures. Humans commit errors for a variety of known and complicated reasons.

4. Latent errors or system failures pose the greatest threat to safety in a complex system because they lead to operator errors. They are failures built into the system and present long before the active error. Latent errors are difficult for the people working in the system to see since they may be hidden in computers or layers of management and people become accustomed to working around the problem.

5. Current responses to errors tend to focus on the active errors. Although this may sometimes be appropriate, in many cases it is not an effec-

tive way to make systems safer. If latent failures remain unaddressed, their accumulation actually makes the system more prone to future failure. Discovering and fixing latent failures and decreasing their duration are likely to have a greater effect on building safer systems than efforts to minimize active errors at the point at which they occur.

6. The application of human factors in other industries has successfully reduced errors. Health care has to look at medical error not as a special case of medicine, but as a special case of error, and to apply the theory and approaches already used in other fields to reduce errors and improve reliability.[56]

REFERENCES

1. Senders, John, "Medical Devices, Medical Errors and Medical Accidents," in *Human Error in Medicine*, ed., Marilyn Sue Bogner, Hillsdale, NJ: Lawrence Erlbaum Associates, 1994.

2. Cook, Richard; Woods, David; Miller, Charlotte, *A Tale of Two Stories: Contrasting Views of Patient Safety*, Chicago: National Patient Safety Foundation, 1998.

3. Cook, Richard and Woods, David, "Operating at the Sharp End: The Complexity of Human Error," in *Human Error in Medicine*, ed., Marilyn Sue Bogner, Hillsdale, NJ: Lawrence Erlbaum Associates, 1994.

4. Perrow, Charles, *Normal Accidents*, New York: Basic Books, 1984.

5. Reason, James, *Human Error*, Cambridge: Cambridge University Press, 1990.

6. Perrow, 1984; Cook and Woods, 1994.

7. Gaba, David M.; Maxwell, Margaret; DeAnda, Abe, Jr.. Anesthetic Mishaps: Breaking the Chain of Accident Evolution. *Anesthesiology*. 66(5):670–676, 1987.

8. Perrow, 1984.

9. Van Cott, Harold, "Human Errors: Their Causes and Reductions," in *Human Error in Medicine*, ed., Marilyn Sue Bogner, Hillsdale, NJ: Lawrence Erlbaum Associates, 1994. Also, Roberts, Karlene, "Organizational Change and A Culture of Safety," in *Proceedings of Enhancing Patient Safety and Reducing Errors in Health Care*, Chicago: National Patient Safety Foundation at the AMA, 1999.

10. Reason, 1990. See also Cook, Woods and Miller, 1998.

11. Norman, Donald, *Things That Make Us Smart, Defending Human Attributes in the Age of Machines,* Menlo Park, CA: Addison-Wesley Publishing Co., 1993.

12. Cooper, Jeffrey B.; Newbower, Ronald; Long, Charlene, et al. Preventable Anesthesia Mishaps: A Study of Human Factors. *Anesthesiology*. 49(6):399–406, 1978.

13. Cooper, Jeffrey B. and Gaba, David M. A Strategy for Preventing Anesthesia Accidents. *International Anesthesia Clinics.* 27(3):148–152, 1989

14. Reason, 1990.

15. Chassin, Mark R.; Galvin, Robert W., and the National Roundtable on Health Care Quality. The Urgent Need to Improve Health Care Quality, *JAMA*. 280(11):1000–1005, 1998.

16. Reason, 1990.

17. Cook, Woods and Miller, 1998.

18. Reason, 1990.

19. Vaughan, Diane, *The Challenger Launch Decision*, Chicago: The University of Chicago Press, 1996.

20. Reason, 1990.

21. Reason, 1990.

22. Roberts, Karlene, 1999. See also: Gaba, David, "Risk, Regulation, Litigation and Organizational Issues in Safety in High-Hazard Industries," position paper for Workshop on Organizational Analysis in High Hazard Production Systems: An Academy/ Industry Dialogue," MIT Endicott House, April 15–18, 1997, NSF Grant No. 9510883-SBR.

23. Sagan, Scott D., *The Limits of Safety*, Princeton, NJ: Princeton University Press, 1993.

24. Sagan, Scott D., 1993 and Robert, Karlene, 1999.

25. Reason, James, "Forward," in *Human Error in Medicine*, ed., Marilyn Sue Bogner, Hillsdale, NJ: Lawrence Erlbaum Associates, 1994.

26. "Agenda for Research and Development in Patient Safety," National Patient Safety Foundation at the AMA, http://www.ama-assn.org/med-sci/npsf/research/research.htm. May 24, 1999.

27. Dye, Kevin M.C.; Post, Diana; Vogt, Eleanor, "Developing a Consensus on the Accountability and Responsibility for the Safe Use of Pharmaceuticals," Preliminary White Paper prepared for the National Patient Safety Foundation, June 1, 1999.

28. Brewer, Timothy; Colditz, Graham A. Postmarketing Surveillance and Adverse Drug Reactions, Current Perspectives and Future Needs. *JAMA.* 281(9):824–829, 1999.

29. *VHA's Patient Safety Improvement Initiative*, presentation to the National Health Policy Forum by Kenneth W. Kizer, Under Secretary for Health, Department of Veterans Affairs, May 14, 1999, Washington, D.C.

30. Leape, Lucian L. Error in Medicine. *JAMA.* 272(23):1851–1857, 1994.

31. Perrow, 1984.

32. Cook and Woods, 1994.

33. Reason. 1990.

34. Norman, 1993.

35. Perrow, 1984.

36. Perrow, 1984.

37. Cook, Woods and Miller, 1998.

38. On the other hand, in some places, the health system may be complex, but loosely coupled. For example, during an emergency, a patient may receive services from a loosely networked set of subsystems—from the ambulance to the emergency room to the outpatient clinic to home care. See Van Cott in Bogner, 1994.

39. Cook and Woods, 1994.

40. Reason, 1990.

41. Reason, 1990.

42. Cook and Woods, 1994.

43. Reason, 1990.

44. Van Cott, 1994.

45. Reason, 1990.

46. Norman, 1993.

47. Cook and Woods, 1994.

48. Van Cott, 1994.

49. Norman, 1993.

50. Institute of Medicine, *Assessing Medical Technologies*, Washington, D.C.: National Academy Press, 1985.

51. Weinger, Matthew B; Pantiskas, Carl; Wiklund, Michael; Carstensen, Peter. Incorporating Human Factors Into the Design of Medical Devices. *JAMA.* 280(17):1484, 1998.

52. Reason, 1990. Leape, 1994.

53. Cooper, Newbower, Long, et al., 1978.

54. Klein, Gary, *Sources of Power: How People Make Decisions*, Cambridge, MA: The MIT Press, 1998.

55. "Current Projects," Human Factors Research and Technology Division, Ames Research Center, NASA, http://human-factors.arc.nasa.gov/frameset.html

56. Senders, 1994.

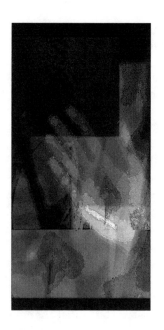

4
Building Leadership and Knowledge for Patient Safety

Errors in the health care industry are at an unacceptably high level. A national commitment to achieve a threshold improvement in patient safety is needed. This will require strong leadership, specification of goals and mechanisms for tracking progress, and an adequate knowledge base. This chapter proposes the development of the Center for Patient Safety within the Agency for Healthcare Research and Quality (AHRQ) to serve as a focal point for these activities. Experience from other industries suggests that unless a Center is created or designated to keep attention focused on patient safety and enhance the base of knowledge and tools, meaningful progress is not likely. Although existing efforts to improve patient safety are valuable, they are inadequate. There is no way of knowing if these efforts are attending to the most critical issues or if they are actually reducing errors. There must be greater attention placed on evaluating current approaches for reducing errors and building new systems to improve patient safety.

RECOMMENDATIONS

RECOMMENDATION 4.1 Congress should create a Center for Patient Safety with the Agency for Healthcare Research and Quality. This Center should

- set the national goals for patient safety, track progress in meeting these goals, and issue an annual report to the President and Congress on patient safety; and
  - develop knowledge and understanding of errors in health care by developing a research agenda, funding Centers of Excellence, evaluating methods for identifying and preventing errors and funding dissemination and communication activities to improve patient safety.

National goals for safety should be established through a process involving consumers, providers, health care organizations, purchasers, researchers, and others. The goals should also reflect areas that represent opportunities for significant improvement. In carrying out its activities in the areas of research and dissemination, the Center for Patient Safety should collaborate with universities, research centers, and various groups involved in education and dissemination, such as the National Patient Safety Foundation.

The committee believes that initial annual funding of $30 to 35 million for a Center for Patient Safety would be appropriate. This initial funding would permit a center to conduct activities in goal setting, tracking, research and dissemination. Funding should grow over time to at least $100 million, or approximately 1% of the $8.8 billion in health care costs attributable to preventable adverse events (see Chapter 2). This level is modest compared to the resources devoted to other major health issues. The committee believes a 50% reduction in errors over five years is imperative.

WHY A CENTER FOR PATIENT SAFETY IS NEEDED

As discussed in Chapter 2, errors in health care are a leading cause of death and injury. Yet, the American public is seemingly unaware of the problem, and the issue is not getting the attention it should from leaders in the health care industry and the professions. Additionally, the knowledge that has been used in other industries to improve safety is rarely applied in health care. Although more needs to be learned, there are actions that can be taken today to improve safety in health care. Medical products can be designed to be safer in use, jobs can be designed to minimize the likelihood of errors, and much can be done to reduce the complexity of care processes.

Although multiple agencies are concerned with selected issues that influence patient safety, there is no focal point for patient safety in health care today. Public- and private-sector oversight organizations, such as state licensure units, accrediting bodies, and federal certification programs devote some attention to patient safety, but patient safety is not their sole focus. The National Patient Safety Foundation conducts educational programs, workshops, and various convening activities but its programs and resources are limited. The Food and Drug Administration (FDA) focuses only on drugs and devices through the regulation of manufacturers. The Joint Commission on Accreditation of Healthcare Organizations' (JCAHO) mission is to improve quality of care through accreditation. This may include issues relevant to patient safety, but patient safety is not its sole focus. Many states operate reporting programs or other oversight programs for patient safety but they take a variety of approaches and focus.

Although anesthesiology applied some of the techniques of system analysis and human factors during the 1980s, the concepts are just beginning to diffuse through the health care industry. The advantage of this lag is that we can learn about building safe systems from the experiences of others. The problem is that there has to be a substantially greater commitment to getting more and better information to advance the science and apply the techniques to health care.

The next section describes how attention to safety issues has been applied in two areas: aviation and occupational health. Both of these examples illustrate how broad-based safety improvements can be accomplished.

HOW OTHER INDUSTRIES HAVE BECOME SAFER

The risk of dying in a domestic jet flight between 1967 and 1976 was 1 in 2 million. By the 1990s, the risk had declined to 1 in 8 million.[1] Between 1970 (when the Occupational Health and Safety Administration was created) and 1996, the workplace death rate was cut in half.[2] Health care has much to learn from other industries about improving safety.

Aviation

Health care is decades behind other industries in terms of creating safer systems. Much of modern safety thinking grew out of military aviation.[3] Until World War II, accidents were viewed primarily as individually caused and safety meant motivating people to "be safe." During the war, generals lost aircraft and pilots in stateside operations and came to realize that planning for safety was as important to the success of a mission as combat planning. System safety continued after the war when several military aviation safety centers were formed in the early 1950s. Human factors started to enter the picture at around the same time. In 1954, the Flight Safety Foundation was formed to design aircraft cockpits using better human engineering. In the mid-1960s, the University of Southern California began its first advanced safety management programs and included a heavy emphasis on human factors. By the 1970s, principles of system safety began to spread to other industries, including rapid rail and the oil industry.

Building on the successful experience and knowledge of military aviation, civilian aviation takes a comprehensive approach to safety, with programs aimed at setting and enforcing standards, accident investigation, incident reporting, and research for continuous improvement.

The Federal Aviation Administration (FAA), housed in the Department of Transportation, has regulatory oversight of the industry and an explicit charge for ensuring safety. Accident investigations are conducted by the National Transportation Safety Board (NTSB), an independent federal agency, which has no regulatory or enforcement power but can issue recommendations to the FAA for regulatory action. Confidential incident reporting (defined as an occurrence associated with the operation of an aircraft that affects or could affect the safety of operations) is conducted through the National Aeronautics and Space Administration Aviation Safety Reporting System (ASRS), which is discussed in Chapter 5.

Research into safety is an integral component of the aviation industry strategy. The national research agenda is set through several mechanisms. First, a formal process determined how to allocate approximately $60 million committed to the Aviation Safety Program for FY 2000 (Cynthia Null, Ames Research Center, personal communication, May 24, 1999). Workshops and meetings were held with multiple agencies and organizations to define the work in the specific program area; participants included NASA, FAA, Department of Defense, all levels of airline employees (pilots, maintenance workers, flight attendants, air traffic controllers), airlines, manufacturers, and others. Existing resources are being redirected consistent with the priorities. Other research that supports safety is funded through "base research" in which in-house researchers propose and carry out research projects for development. Research into human factors is part of the base research program.

The Aviation Safety Reporting System may also conduct "topical research," which could include structured callback studies on a certain topic or basic research. This area of work is funded within ASRS's main program, but funding is not often available (Linda Connell, Director of ASRS, personal communication, May 20, 1999). Human factors researchers at Ames may also tap into the ASRS database to generate hypotheses which can then be tested through other research.

Finally, the FAA itself maintains several databases that aggregate a variety of statistics (e.g., airline operations such as departures, hours and miles flown, history of safety recommendations to different parts of the industry and responses to them). FAA and NASA coordinate their research efforts to minimize duplication. For example, both agencies may jointly contribute to a single effort, or they may fund different, but complementary, aspects of an issue.

Charles Billings, M.D., designer and founder of the Aviation Safety Reporting System, has stated his belief that aviation would not be as safe as it is today without the FAA.[4] By setting standards, maintaining multiple databases to monitor trends, and supporting research to constantly improve systems, the FAA (in collaboration with other agencies such as NASA and NTSB) has made flying safer.

Occupational Health

The Occupational Safety and Health Act of 1970 created both the Occupational Safety and Health Administration (OSHA), housed in the Department of Labor, and its research arm, the National Institute for Occupational Safety and Health (NIOSH), housed in the Centers for Disease Control and Prevention (CDC) in the Department of Health and Human Services. OSHA's purpose is to encourage employers and employees to reduce workplace hazards and to implement new, or improve existing, safety and health programs. It provides for research in occupational health and safety, maintains reporting and record-keeping systems, establishes training programs, and develops and enforces mandatory standards for job safety and health.[5] OSHA is administered through a combined federal–state approach. States that develop their own programs and have an approved plan receive up to 50 percent of the plan's approved operating costs.

OSHA requires employers with 11 or more employees to routinely maintain records of occupational injury and illness as they occur. These records are not submitted to OSHA, but must be made available during inspection and shared with OSHA if the company is selected for an annual tracking survey. OSHA and the Bureau of Labor and Statistics both conduct sample surveys to collect the routine data maintained by companies. These surveys are used to construct population rates or to examine particular issues of concern.

A related incentive for employers to create a safe environment is the worker's compensation program. Under state law, employers must pay the premium for insuring workers against the medical costs of injuries sustained while on the job. Responsibility for the costs associated with workers compensation further encourages employers to improve the safety systems in their companies.

Responsibility for research and for identifying new safety improvements is housed in a separate agency. The National Institute for Occupational Safety and Health (NIOSH) has the responsibility for conducting research and making recommendations for the prevention of work-related illnesses and injuries.[6] It conducts and funds research on safety and health problems, provides technical assistance to OSHA, and recommends standards for OSHA adoption. Although OSHA provides input into the NIOSH research agenda, it is set mainly through input from other stakeholders, including company requests. Information gathered by NIOSH from these companies for research purposes is not shared with OSHA for regulatory purposes.

A major agenda for research was established in 1996 through the National Occupational Research Agenda (NORA). Input was obtained from 500 public and private organizations to provide a framework for safety research during the next decade and to guide intramural and extramural funding decisions. Twenty-one research priorities were selected and are now being implemented, mostly by shifting existing resources so that over time, more monies are directed to the priority areas. For example, in 1998, NIOSH and three institutes at the National Institutes of Health (NIH) committed $24 million over three years to certain priority areas.[7] For 1999, NIOSH's operating budget is $200 million, of which $156 million is for intramural and extramural research projects (Janice Klink, Associate Director for Policy, Planning, and Legislation, NIOSH, personal communication, May 19, 1999).

Lessons Learned

There are several key points to be taken from the experiences in aviation and occupational health. In each of these areas, there was a growing awareness of safety concerns and the need to improve performance. This led to comprehensive strategies, which included the creation of a national focal point for leadership, development of a knowledge base, and dissemination of information throughout the industry.

In both areas, there is a designated government agency with regulatory responsibility for safety, which is separate from the agency responsible for research. Although the entity responsible for research may generate reports that are useful to the regulatory authority in setting standards, data and information collected from organizations are not available for use in enforcing standards on a particular organization.

Both areas recognized the need to rapidly expand the knowledge base on safety and to establish ongoing processes for the diffusion of this knowledge. The creation of a carefully constructed research agenda was developed with broad-based input from the industry and is implemented through both public- and private-sector programs to draw upon the best expertise in the academic and scientific communities.

Finally, substantial resources were devoted to these initiatives. Achieving steady improvement requires that adequate resources be sustained over a sufficient period of time. The safety improvements did not occur because of a one-time effort. The results were achieved through an ongoing commitment of resources and leadership.

Although some of these components can be found in health care today—regulatory oversight, research and dissemination—there is no cohesive effort to improve safety in health care, and the resources devoted to enhancing and disseminating the knowledge base are wholly inadequate. Given the experience of other industries, health care is not likely to make significant safety improvements without a more comprehensive, coordinated approach.

OPTIONS FOR ESTABLISHING A CENTER FOR PATIENT SAFETY

Objectives

The objectives of a Center for Patient Safety are to provide leadership for safety improvements throughout the industry, to establish goals and track progress in achieving results, and to expand the knowledge base for improving safety in health care.

A central objective of the Center for Patient Safety is to provide visibility to safety concerns. The leadership of the Center must possess the requisite expertise and stature to communicate with a broad audience to raise awareness of safety concerns and convene stakeholders to identify strategies for improving safety.

Expanding the knowledge base requires the formulation and implementation of a research agenda. Such an agenda should include short-term, focused studies as well as long-term, population studies. Expanding the knowledge base also requires effective methods for diffusing the new knowledge to a variety of audiences, including those in the industry and the general public.

The Center should develop a limited number of high-priority goals based on careful analysis of areas in which improvements will result in the greatest gains in terms of reduced morbidity and mortality and reduced costs. Specific goals identify priority areas for the industry so the industry can respond supportively. Specific goals also provide a basis for tracking change. Safety efforts must be evaluated to determine whether actual improvements are being achieved and to ensure that resources are allocated to high-priority areas that will have the most impact on patients.

Implementation Options

The committee believes that an organization designated as the focal point for patient safety should have the following characteristics. First, it should be involved in a broader agenda for improving quality. Patient safety is part of general quality improvement, even if certain safety problems may utilize distinct knowledge and expertise. It would not be desirable to have one agency focused on quality issues and a separate agency focused on patient safety.

Second, the agency should possess the core competencies required to undertake the broad array of tasks identified. Although some may be carried out through partnership arrangements, the agency should have adequate expertise and funding to engage in strategic planning, convening, tracking, research and evaluation, and information dissemination activities.

Finally, the designated agency should be able to work collaboratively with other health- and non-health-related safety agencies. For example, it should consult with NTSB and ASRS to understand how an entire industry sets safety as a priority and becomes safer over time. Experts from OSHA may also offer guidance on their experience in encouraging companies to build safety systems within their own organizations. Collaboration with the National Patient Safety Foundation might be desirable in carrying out various agenda-setting and education activities.

The committee discussed three alternative organizational arrangements for a Center for Patient Safety. One option considered was the creation of a new, free-standing agency whose sole purpose is to focus on patient safety issues. A second alternative was to place such a center within NIH, as a defined division or institute. A third option was to place the proposed Center for Patient Safety within the AHRQ.

The committee decided that placing the Center within AHRQ was the best option for several reasons. Although a dedicated agency might be most able to maintain a focus on patient safety, this option should be pursued as a last resort, given the resources and time required to establish a new agency. NIH has the expertise and industry respect to drive a basic research agenda and has built partnerships with other agencies, but its agenda is already very broad and does not routinely involve analyses of systems of care or quality measurement or improvement.

AHRQ is already involved with a broad range of quality-of-care issues, including quality measurement, quality improvement, and identification of best practices. The Consumer Assessment of Health Plans (CAHPS) is a standardized measurement and reporting tool in which consumers report their experience with specific aspects of their health plans to assess the features that form the basis of overall satisfaction. The goal is to provide consumers and purchasers with objective information for choosing among health plans. Another initiative is the support of evidence-based practice centers. These are five-year contracts awarded to 12 institutions to review scientific literature on assigned clinical care topics and to produce evidence reports and technology assessments, conduct research on methodologies and the effectiveness of their implementation, and participate in technical assistance activities.

AHRQ also is engaged in activities specifically related to patient safety, and these activities constitute a good base of experience upon which to expand. AHRQ has sponsored research in the area of patient safety, specifically in the areas of medication errors, diagnostic inaccuracies, inaccurate information recall by patients, and system failures in adverse drug events.[8] A recent Memorandum of Understanding was executed with the National Institutes on Aging to cofund a grant to examine adverse drug events among a geriatric population in an ambulatory setting. Technologies tested in AHRQ-sponsored research that would improve patient safety include computerized monitoring of adverse drug events, computer-generated reminders for follow-up testing, standardized protocols, and computer-assisted decision making.

A new AHRQ endeavor initiated in 1998 is the establishment of Centers for Education and Research in Therapeutics (CERTs). CERTs will conduct research to increase understanding of ways to improve the appropriate and effective use of pharmaceuticals and other interventions to avoid adverse drug events. CERTs will also increase knowledge of the possible risks of new drugs and combinations of drugs, as they are prescribed in everyday practice. CERTs are being implemented in collaboration with FDA.[9]

AHRQ also has experience in collaborating with other relevant organizations. It has provided support for meetings on patient safety and is a member of the National Patient Safety Partnership, a public–private group dedicated to reducing preventable adverse medical events. AHRQ participates in the Quality Interagency Coordinating Committee (QuIC), which is developing an initiative on reducing medical errors. AHRQ also sponsors the User Liaison Program (ULP) as a vehicle to link states, local health policy makers and researchers to disseminate research to states, conduct workshops, and provide technical assistance.[10]

Finally, the agency's reauthorization legislation for FY 2000 is expected to include explicit language defining a focus on reducing medical errors and improving patient safety.

FUNCTIONS OF THE CENTER FOR PATIENT SAFETY

Creating an information infrastructure and building a better evidence base for patient safety are critical to taking a more strategic approach to reducing medical errors and improving patient safety. The goal is to improve decision making by policy makers, regulators, health care organizations, and others, so that decisions are based on evidence rather than anecdote. Good information can and should be used to guide the development and continuous improvement of standards and to support communication and outreach efforts.

The Center for Patient Safety should build an information infrastructure and resource for patient safety. It should have a broad agenda comprised of multiple programs. In its first five full years of existence, it should deliver the following products:

1. Establish a limited set of high-priority goals for improving patient safety based on expert opinion and review of the evidence on errors.

2. Assess progress toward national goals by compiling aggregate information from state adverse event reporting systems, voluntary reporting systems, health care organizations, and other sources; and periodically conducting a representative survey of health care organizations.

3. Develop a research agenda, conduct and fund intramural and extra-

mural research to assess the magnitude of errors, and the role of human factors, and test and evaluate approaches for preventing errors.

4. Define feasible prototype systems (best practices) and tools for safety in key processes, including both clinical and managerial support systems for:

- medication systems (from prescribing to administering),
- operating rooms and surgery processes,
- emergency departments,
- management of diagnostic tests, screening, and information,
- intensive care units,
- neonatal intensive care units,
- care of frail elderly (e.g., falls, decubitus, etc.),
- the use of simulation and simulators in health care, and
- team training and crew resource management applications in health care.

5. Develop instructional methods, demonstration projects, and technical support to ensure widespread implementation of the prototype systems and tools identified above.

6. Conduct periodic evaluations of error reporting systems for two purposes: assessing the impact of mandatory reporting systems in various states and identifying best practices in program design and implementation; and assessing the usefulness of voluntary reporting systems in identifying important safety improvements and determining whether current levels of participation by health care organizations are adequate or additional incentives are needed.

7. Provide support to health care organizations for internal quality improvement demonstration projects to prevent and reduce errors.

8. Develop tools and methods for educating consumers about patient safety.

9. Issue an annual report on progress made to improve patient safety, and recommend changes for continuously improving patient safety to appropriate parties, such as FDA, states, accrediting agencies, professional associations, group purchasers, and health care organizations.

In setting the research agenda, the Center for Patient Safety should establish a formal process to gather input on priorities, methodologies and approaches for research. Advice should be obtained from a wide range of people and organizations who will use and can benefit from the availability of information. It should look at the experiences of other industries and the processes they employed, such as aviation and occupational health, as already described. Initial areas for attention might include the following:

• enhance understanding of the impact of various management practices (e.g., maximum work hours and overtime) on the likelihood of errors;
• apply safety methods and technologies from other industries to health care, especially human factors and engineering principles;
• increase understanding of errors in different settings (e.g., ambulatory or home care) and for vulnerable populations (e.g., children, elderly);
• establish baseline rates of specific types of errors and monitor trends;
• monitor error rates that accompany the introduction of new technologies; and
• increase understanding of the use of information technology to improve patient safety (e.g., automated drug order or entry systems, reminder systems).

In conducting research and developing prototype systems, the Center should consider providing support for the establishment of several Centers of Excellence in academic or applied research settings and which can gather expertise from diverse settings as needed. Centers of Excellence might focus on particular types of errors (e.g., medication-related errors), errors in particular settings or clinical specialties (e.g., intensive care), or types of interventions or strategies that might be applied across many areas and settings (e.g., interdisciplinary teams).

In establishing Centers of Excellence, the Center for Patient Safety will want to learn from and coordinate with the Veterans Health Administration (VHA), which has pursued a similar strategy on a much smaller scale. As part of its comprehensive program in improving patient safety throughout their delivery system, the Veterans Health Administration has committed $6 million to establish four Patient Safety Centers of Inquiry, focused on researching new knowledge in patient safety, with special emphasis on transferring safety technologies from other high-risk industries to health care, and on disseminating existing knowledge.[11]

It is also imperative that the Center for Patient Safety focus adequate attention on the communication of information on and knowledge of patient safety. The support and production of more and better information on medical errors and patient safety will be of little use without explicit mechanisms identified for dissemination of the information and recommended actions. Although dissemination of information is sometimes an afterthought, there are attributes that can improve outreach. Important factors that have been identified are translating raw data into summary measures and information that can be used; presenting information in formats that are tailored to different audiences; and providing multiple ways to access the information, such as print, television, radio, videotaped presentations, online services, and face-to-face presentations. The information also needs to be timely and to come from a credible source.[12]

At the present time, there are few objective sources for the latest information on patient safety. Improvements may be made in practice within health care organizations, but there is no way to disseminate such information to a broader audience. An important responsibility of the Center for Patient Safety should be to work to increase the frequency of communication about patient safety to multiple audiences. In carrying out its responsibilities to communicate information and knowledge on safety, the Center should work closely with existing organizations that have related objectives, including public and private organizations; policy, educational and accrediting entities; and quality oversight organizations.

The National Patient Safety Foundation (NPSF) is an existing organization that may be able to serve this resource and dissemination role. The National Patient Safety Foundation was formed by the American Medical Association in 1997 as an independent, nonprofit research and education organization, whose mission is to improve patient safety in the delivery of care. The AMA's goal was to establish linkages with other health care organizations dedicated to improving patient safety.

NPSF is well positioned to "translate" concerns and findings about patient safety between many different parties because of the broad base of representation on its board that can communicate with various constituencies and its proven ability to convene a mix of stakeholders. NPSF's core strategies include activities to raise awareness and foster communication and dialogue to enhance patient safety and to develop information, collaborative relationships, and educational approaches that advance patient safety.[13] It supports an annual grant program for innovative research to prevent patient injuries; has conducted a benchmark survey to capture consumer attitudes, experience and expectations about health care safety; conducts regional forums to bring together community and health leaders in local communities and convenes national conferences that brings together leaders in patient safety from around the world.[14] NPSF has also begun developing a clearinghouse function to collect patient safety information that can be accessed by both health professionals and consumers.

The National Patient Safety Partnership is a voluntary public–private partnership, comprised of the American Hospital Association, American

Medical Association (AMA), American Nurses Association, Association of American Medical Colleges, JCAHO, National Patient Safety Foundation of the AMA, and Department of Veterans Affairs as charter members. Additional members include AHRQ, FDA, HCFA, NIOSH, and the Department of Defense, Health Affairs. Its primary concerns have focused on year 2000 (Y2K) issues and adverse drug events.[15]

The deliverables previously identified for the Center for Patient Safety include the development of tools and methods for educating consumers about patient safety. Although consumers are an important audience, there are many other constituencies that must be reached, including health professionals and managers, health care organizations, state and national policy makers, regulators, pharmaceutical companies and medical device manufacturers, professional groups and associations, medical and health care training centers, and various forms of media. Although AHRQ and the Center for Patient Safety will disseminate their work on patient safety through current mechanisms (e.g., reports, newsletters, Internet), the NPSF and the National Patient Safety Partnership are existing organizations that can support a broad approach for dissemination activities.

RESOURCES REQUIRED FOR A CENTER FOR PATIENT SAFETY

In determining what would be an adequate level of funding for a Center for Patient Safety, the committee considered three things: (1) research investments made to address health care issues of a similar magnitude; (2) investments in safety research in other industries; and (3) operating budgets for research initiatives with similar programs.

The United States invests significant resources in research to reduce the morbidity and mortality associated with various diseases and health concerns. As noted in Chapter 2, medical errors among hospitalized patients ranks as a leading cause of death, exceeding the number of deaths in 1997 due to motor vehicle accidents, breast cancer, or AIDS. NIH funding in 1998 for AIDS was estimated at $1.6 billion and for breast cancer, $433 million.[16] Another funding comparison in health care is to examine research centers that have a more focused agenda. The National Institute for Deafness and Other Communication Disorders has funding of approximately $230 million in FY99.[17] The National Institute of Nursing Research received funding of approximately $63 million in FY99.[18] These are examples of "smaller" institutes at NIH.

The success of other industries in improving safety is undoubtedly attributable in part to the commitment made to enhancing the knowledge base. As noted previously, the NIOSH operating budget for 1999 is $200 million, of which $156 million is for intramural and extramural research projects. The Aviation Safety Program at NASA Ames Research Center allocated approximately $60 million for FY 2000.

Another funding comparison is the resources devoted by AHRQ to different programs. In FY 1999, $2 million was appropriated for the CERTs, newly established research centers; twice that amount is expected for FY 2000 to continue funding.[19] The Evidence-Based Practice Centers at AHRQ are funded at more than $3 million per year (Nancy Foster, AHRQ, personal communication, July 22, 1999). AHRQ also conducts a Medical Expenditure Panel Survey for which almost $35 million was appropriated in FY 1999.[20]

Finally, the Veterans Health Administration created several centers within its own system devoted to research and improved understanding about medical errors. It committed $6 million over 4 years.

Initial annual funding of $30 to 35 million for the Center for Patient Safety would be reasonable. This estimate is based on the functions that the center is to perform. Goal setting would involve convening a broad set of audiences for input into goals and a research agenda. Regional meetings and other mechanisms may be employed to gather input. It is estimated that approximately $2 million would be needed for goal setting activities. Tracking progress on meeting goals would require periodic data collection from health care organizations. The Harvard Medical Practice Study reviewed over 31,000 hospital records and cost approximately $3 million. The development and implementation of a national survey is estimated at $5 million. To implement a research agenda, it is estimated that five Centers of Excellence would be formed, each with a specific focus of attention. Each Center of Excellence should be initially funded at $5 million, growing over time to $15 million each. Dissemination of information to the industry, general public, policy makers and others is estimated initially at $5 million. The estimate of initial funding seems modest in light of the investments made to address health concerns of similar magnitude.

The committee believes that the growth in the funding level is necessary to communicate to researchers, states, professional groups and health care organizations that this will be a sustained effort. In the absence of a significant long term commitment to funding, researchers are unlikely to re-orient their focus to patient safety. The patient safety initiatives of other groups, such as states, professional associations and health care organizations are likely to be far more successful if accompanied by a steady flow of new knowledge, tools, and prototype systems. It can take several years to create awareness about safety and build interest. The growth in funding recognizes that initial funding should be at a lower, but sufficient, level to begin work in the area, but should grow over time as the efforts evolve and expand.

REFERENCES

1. "The Aviation Safety System," Aviation Safety Information From The Federal Aviation Administration, http:www.faa.gov/publicinfo.htm

2. "Common Sense at Work," OSHA Vital Facts 1997, Occupational Safety and Health Administration, Department of Labor, http://www.osha-slc.gov/OshDoc/OSHFacts/OSHAFacts.html, last modified May 4, 1999.

3. Miller, C.O., "System Safety," in *Human Factors in Aviation*, eds., Earl L. Wiener, David C. Nagel, San Diego, CA: Academic Press, Inc., 1988.

4. Comments to Subcommittee on Creating an External Environment for Quality, IOM Quality of Health Care in America project, January 28, 1999.

5. "All About OSHA," OSHA 2056, 1995 (Revised), http://www.osha.gov

6. "About NIOSH," National Institute for Occupational Safety and Health, Centers for Disease Control, http://www.cdc.gov/niosh/about.html

7. "NIOSH/NORA Fact Sheet, July 1999," www.cdc.gov/niosh/99-130.html, July 29, 1999.

8. *Reducing Errors in Health Care*. Research in Action, September, 1998. Agency for Healthcare Research and Quality, Rockville, MD. http://www.AHRQ.gov/research/errors.htm.

9. *Therapeutics Research Centers to be Established Through Federal Cooperative Agreement Funding: Applications Sought*. Press Release. February 1, 1999. Agency for Healthcare Research and Quality, Rockville, MD. http://www.AHRQ.gov/news/press/pre1999/certspr.htm.

10. "Research Findings, User Liaison Program," http://www.AHRQ.gov/research.

11. *NPSF News Brief*, No. 6, March 22, 1999, The National Patient Safety Foundation at the AMA. http://www.ama-assn.org/med-sci/npsf/news/03_22_99.htm.

12. *Quality First: Better Health Care for All Americans*, The President's Advisory Commission on Consumer Protection and Quality in the Health Care Industry. Final Report, Washington, D.C., March 1998.

13. *Request for Proposals for Research in Patient Safety*, The National Patient Safety Foundation at the AMA. http://www.ama-assn.org/med-sci/npsf/focus.htm, January 1999.

14. "Leading the Way," National Patient Safety Foundation at the AMA, http://www.ama-assn.org/med-sci/npsf/broc.htm.

15. Kenneth W. Kizer, presentation at National Health Policy Forum, May 14, 1999, Washington, D.C.

16. Institute of Medicine, Scientific Opportunities and Public Needs. Improving Priority Setting and Public Input at the National Institutes of Health. Washington, D.C.: National Academy Press, 1998.

17. "Fiscal Year 2000 President's Budget request for the National Institute on Deaf-

ness and Other Communication Disorders," Statement by Dr. James F. Battey, Jr., Director, National Institute of Deafness and Other Communication Disorders, www.nih.nidcd/about/director/openstate00.htm

18. Fiscal Year 2000 President's Budget request for the National Institute of Nursing Research," Statement by Dr. Patricia A. Grady, Director, National Institute on Nursing Research, www.nih.gov/ninr/openingstatement99.htm.

19. Margaret Keyes, AHRQ Center for Quality Measurement and Improvement, presentation to Subcommittee on Creating an External Environment for Quality of the IOM Quality of Care in America Study, June 15, 1999.

20. *Justification for Budget Estimates for Appropriations Committees, Fiscal Year 2000.* Agency for Healthcare Research and Quality, Rockville, MD. http://www.AHRQ.gov/news/cj2000/cjweb00.htm.

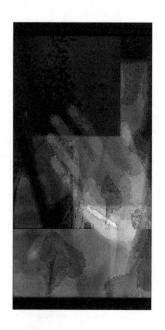

5
Error
Reporting
Systems

Although the previous chapter talked about creating and disseminating new knowledge to prevent errors from ever happening, this chapter looks at what happens after an error occurs and how to learn from errors and prevent their recurrence. One way to learn from errors is to establish a reporting system. Reporting systems have the potential to serve two important functions. They can hold providers accountable for performance or, alternatively, they can provide information that leads to improved safety. Conceptually, these purposes are not incompatible, but in reality, they can prove difficult to satisfy simultaneously.

Reporting systems whose primary purpose is to hold providers accountable are "mandatory reporting systems." Reporting focuses on errors associated with serious injuries or death. Most mandatory reporting systems are operated by state regulatory programs that have the authority to investigate specific cases and issue penalties or fines for wrong-doing. These systems serve three purposes. First, they provide the public with a minimum level of protection by assuring that the most serious errors are reported and investigated and appropriate follow-up action is taken. Second, they provide an incentive to health care organizations to improve patient safety in order to avoid the potential penalties and public exposure. Third, they require all health care organizations to make some level of investment in patient safety, thus creating a more level playing field. While safety experts recognize that errors resulting in serious harm are the "tip of the iceberg," they represent the small subset of errors that signal major system breakdowns with grave consequences for patients.

Reporting systems that focus on safety improvement are "voluntary reporting systems." The focus of voluntary systems is usually on errors that resulted in no harm (sometimes referred to as "near misses") or very minimal patient harm. Reports are usually submitted in confidence outside of the public arena and no penalties or fines are issued around a specific case. When voluntary systems focus on the analysis of "near misses," their aim is to identify and remedy vulnerabilities in systems before the occurrence of harm. Voluntary reporting systems are particularly useful for identifying types of errors that occur too infrequently for an individual health care organization to readily detect based on their own data, and patterns of errors that point to systemic issues affecting all health care organizations.

The committee believes that there is a need for both mandatory and voluntary reporting systems and that they should be operated separately. Mandatory reporting systems should focus on detection of errors that result in serious patient harm or death (i.e., preventable adverse events). Adequate attention and resources must be devoted to analyzing reports and taking appropriate follow-up action to hold health care organizations accountable. The results of analyses of individual reports should be made available to the public.

The continued development of voluntary reporting efforts should also be encouraged. As discussed in Chapter 6, reports submitted to voluntary reporting systems should be afforded legal protections from data discoverability. Health care organizations should be encouraged to participate in voluntary reporting systems as an important component of their patient safety programs.

For either type of reporting program, implementation without adequate resources for analysis and follow-up will not be useful. Receiving reports is only the first step in the process of reducing errors. Sufficient attention must be devoted to analyzing and understanding the causes of errors in order to make improvements.

RECOMMENDATIONS

RECOMMENDATION 5.1 A nationwide mandatory reporting system should be established that provides for the collection of standardized information by state governments about adverse events that result in death or serious harm. Reporting should initially be required

of hospitals and eventually be required of other institutional and ambulatory care delivery settings. Congress should

- designate the National Forum for Health Care Quality Measurement and Reporting as the entity responsible for promulgating and maintaining a core set of reporting standards to be used by states, including a nomenclature and taxonomy for reporting;
- require all health care organizations to report standardized information on a defined list of adverse events;
- provide funds and technical expertise for state governments to establish or adapt their current error reporting systems to collect the standardized information, analyze it and conduct follow-up action as needed with health care organizations. Should a state choose not to implement the mandatory reporting system, the Department of Health and Human Services should be designated as the responsible entity; and designate the Center for Patient Safety to:

(1)   convene states to share information and expertise, and to evaluate alternative approaches taken for implementing reporting programs, identify best practices for implementation, and assess the impact of state programs; and
(2)   receive and analyze aggregate reports from states to identify persistent safety issues that require more intensive analysis and/or a broader-based response (e.g., designing prototype systems or requesting a response by agencies, manufacturers or others).

Mandatory reporting systems should focus on the identification of serious adverse events attributable to error. Adverse events are deaths or serious injuries resulting from a medical intervention.[1] Not all, but many, adverse events result from errors. Mandatory reporting systems generally require health care organizations to submit reports on all serious adverse events for two reasons: they are easy to identify and hard to conceal. But it is only after careful analysis that the subset of reports of particular interest, namely those attributable to error, are identified and follow-up action can be taken.

The committee also believes that the focus of mandatory reporting system should be narrowly defined. There are significant costs associated with reporting systems, both costs to health care organizations and the cost of operating the oversight program. Furthermore, reporting is useful only if it includes analysis and follow-up of reported events. A more narrowly defined program has a better chance of being successful.

A standardized reporting format is needed to define what ought to be reported and how it should be reported. There are three purposes to having a standardized format. First, a standardized format permits data to be combined and tracked over time. Unless there are consistent definitions and methods for data collection across organizations, the data cannot be aggregated. Second, a standardized format lessens the burden on health care organizations that operate in multiple states or are subject to reporting requirements of multiple agencies and/or private oversight processes and group purchasers. Third, a standardized format facilitates communication with consumers and purchasers about patient safety.

The recently established National Forum for Health Care Quality Measurement and Reporting is well positioned to play a lead role in promulgating standardized reporting formats, including a nomenclature and taxonomy for reporting. The Forum is a public/private partnership charged with developing a comprehensive quality measurement and public reporting strategy. The existing reporting systems (i.e., national and state programs, public and private sector programs) also represent a growing body of expertise on how to collect and analyze information about errors, and should be consulted during this process.[2]

RECOMMENDATION 5.2 The development of voluntary reporting efforts should be encouraged. The Center for Patient Safety should

- **describe and disseminate information on existing voluntary reporting programs to encourage greater participation in them and track the development of new reporting systems as they form;**
- **convene sponsors and users of external reporting systems to evaluate what works and what does not work well in the programs, and ways to make them more effective;**
- **periodically assess whether additional efforts are needed to address gaps in information to improve patient safety and to encourage health care organizations to participate in voluntary reporting programs; and**
- **fund and evaluate pilot projects for reporting systems, both within individual health care organizations and collaborative efforts among health care organizations.**

Voluntary reporting systems are an important part of an overall program for improving patient safety and should be encouraged. Accrediting bodies and group purchasers should recognize and reward health care organizations that participate in voluntary reporting systems. The existing voluntary systems vary in scope, type of information collected, confidentiality provisions, how feedback to reporters is fashioned, and what is done with the information received in the reports. Although one of the voluntary medication error reporting systems has been in operation for 25 years, others have evolved in just the past six years. A concerted analysis should assess which features make the reporting system most useful, and how the systems can be made more effective and complementary.

The remainder of this chapter contains a discussion of existing error reporting systems, both within health care and other industries, and a discussion of the committee's recommendations.

REVIEW OF EXISTING REPORTING SYSTEMS IN HEALTH CARE

There are a number of reporting systems in health care and other industries. The existing programs vary according to a number of design features. Some programs mandate reporting, whereas others are voluntary. Some programs receive reports from individuals, while others receive reports from organizations. The advantage of receiving reports from organizations is that it signifies that the institution has some commitment to making corrective system changes. The advantage of receiving reports from individuals is the opportunity for input from frontline practitioners. Reporting systems can also vary in their scope. Those that currently exist in health care tend to be more narrow in focus (e.g., medication-related error), but there are examples outside health care of very comprehensive systems.

There appear to be three general approaches taken in the existing reporting systems. One approach involves mandatory reporting to an external entity. This approach is typically employed by states that require reporting by health care organizations for purposes of accountability. A second approach is voluntary, confidential reporting to an external group for purposes of quality improvement (the first model may also use the information for quality improvement, but that is not its main purpose). There are medication reporting programs that fall into this category. Voluntary reporting systems are also used extensively in other industries such as aviation. The third approach is mandatory internal reporting with audit. For example, the Occupational Safety and Health Administration (OSHA) requires organizations to keep data internally according to a standardized format and to make the data available during on-site inspections. The data maintained internally are not routinely submitted, but may be submitted if the organization is selected in the sample of an annual survey.

The following sections provide an overview of existing health care reporting systems in these categories. They also include two examples from areas outside health care. The Aviation Safety Reporting System is discussed because it represents the most sophisticated and long-standing voluntary external reporting system. It differs from the voluntary external reporting systems in health care because of its comprehensive scope. Since there are currently no examples of mandatory internal reporting with audit, the characteristics of the OSHA approach are described.

Mandatory External Reporting

State Adverse Event Tracking

In a recent survey of states conducted by the Joint Commission on Accreditation of Healthcare Organizations (JCAHO), it was found that at least one-third of states have some form of adverse event reporting system.[3] It is likely that the actual percentage is higher because not all states responded to the survey and some of the nonrespondents may have reporting requirements. During the development of this report, the Institute of Medicine (IOM) interviewed 13 states with reporting systems to learn more about the scope and operation of their programs. The remainder of this section relates to information provided to the IOM. Appendix D summarizes selected characteristics of the reporting systems in these states, and includes information on what is reported to the state, who is required to submit reports, the number of reports received in the most recent year available, when the program began, who has access to the information collected and how the state uses the information that is obtained. This is not intended as a comprehensive review, but rather, as an overview of how some state reporting systems are designed.

States have generally focused their reporting systems on patient injuries or facility issues (e.g., fire, structural issues). Reports are submitted by health care organizations, mostly hospitals and/or nursing homes, although some states also include ambulatory care centers and other licensed facilities. Although the programs may require reporting from a variety of licensed facilities, nursing homes often consume a great deal of state regulatory attention. In Connecticut, 14,000 of almost 15,000 reports received in 1996 were from nursing homes.

Several of the programs have been in place for ten years or longer, although they have undergone revisions since their inception. For example,

New York State's program has been in place since 1985, but it has been reworked three times, the most recent version having been implemented in 1998 after a three-year pilot test.

Underreporting is believed to plague all programs, especially in their early years of operation. Colorado's program received 17 reports in its first two years of operation,[4] but ten years later, received more than 1000 reports. On the other hand, New York's program receives approximately 20,000 reports annually.

The state programs reported that they protected the confidentiality of certain data, but policies varied. Patient identifiers were never released; practitioner's identity was rarely available. States varied in whether or not the hospital's name was released. For example, Florida is barred from releasing any information with hospital or patient identification; it releases only a statewide summary.

The submission of a report itself did not trigger any public release of information. Some states posted information on the Internet, but only after the health department took official action against the facility. New York has plans to release hospital-specific aggregate information (e.g., how many reports were submitted), but no information on any specific report.

Few states aggregate the data or analyze them to identify general trends. For the most part, analysis and follow-up occurs on a case-by-case basis. For example, in some states, the report alerted the health department to a problem; the department would assess whether or not to conduct a follow-up inspection of the facility. If an inspection was conducted, the department might require corrective action and/or issue a deficiency notice for review during application for relicensure.

Two major impediments to making greater use of the reported data were identified: lack of resources and limitations in data. Many states cited a lack of resources as a reason for conducting only limited analysis of data. Several states had, or were planning to construct a database so that information could be tracked over time but had difficulty getting the resources or expertise to do so. Additionally, several states indicated that the information they received in reports from health care organizations was inadequate and variable. The need for more standardized reporting formats was noted.

A focus group was convened with representatives from approximately 20 states at the 12th Annual conference of the National Academy of State Health Policy (August 2, 1999). This discussion reinforced the concerns heard in IOM's telephone interviews. Resource constraints were identified, as well as the need for tools, methods, and protocols to constructively address the issue. The group also identified the need for mechanisms to improve the flow of information between the state, consumers, and providers to encourage safety and quality improvements. The need for collaboration across states to identify and promote best practices was also highlighted. Finally, the group emphasized the need to create greater awareness of the problem of patient safety and errors in health care among the general public and among health care professionals as well.

In summary, the state programs appear to provide a public response for investigation of specific events,[5] but are less successful in synthesizing information to analyze where broad system improvements might take place or in communicating alerts and concerns to other institutions. Resource constraints and, in some cases, poorly specified reporting requirements contribute to the inability to have as great an impact as desired.

Food and Drug Administration (FDA)

Reports submitted to FDA are one part of the surveillance system for monitoring adverse events associated with medical products after their approval (referred to as postmarketing surveillance).[6] Reports may be submitted directly to FDA or through MedWatch, FDA's reporting program. For medical devices, manufacturers are required to report deaths, serious injuries, and malfunctions to FDA. User facilities (hospitals, nursing homes) are required to report deaths to the manufacturer and FDA and to report serious injuries to the manufacturer. For suspected adverse events associated with drugs, reporting is mandatory for manufacturers and voluntary for physicians, consumers, and others. FDA activities are discussed in greater detail in Chapter 7.

Voluntary External Reporting

Joint Commission on Accreditation of Healthcare Organizations (JCAHO)

JCAHO initiated a sentinel event reporting system for hospitals in 1996 (see Chapter 7 for a discussion on JCAHO activities related to accreditation). For its program, a sentinel event is defined as an "unexpected occurrence or variation involving death or serious physical or psychological injury or the risk thereof." Sentinel events subject to reporting are those that have resulted in an unanticipated death or major permanent loss of function not related to the natural course of the patient's illness or underlying condition, or an event that meets one of the following criteria (even if the outcome was not death or major permanent loss of function): suicide of a patient in a setting where the patient receives around-the-clock care; infant abduction or discharge to the wrong facility; rape; hemolytic transfusion reaction involving administration of blood or blood products having major blood group incompatibilities; or surgery on the wrong patient or wrong body part.[7]

The Joint Commission requires that an organization experiencing a sentinel event conduct a root cause analysis, a process for identifying the basic or causal factors of the event. A hospital may voluntarily report an incident to JCAHO and submit their root cause analysis (including actions for improvement). If an organization experiences a sentinel event but does not voluntarily report it and JCAHO discovers the event (e.g., from the media, patient report, employee report), the organization is still required to prepare an acceptable root cause analysis and action plan. If the root cause analysis and action plan are not acceptable, the organization may be placed on accreditation watch until an acceptable plan is prepared. Root cause analyses and action plans are confidential; they are destroyed after required data elements have been entered into a JCAHO database to be used for tracking and sharing risk reduction strategies.

JCAHO encountered some resistance from hospitals when it introduced the sentinel event reporting program and is still working through the issues today. Since the initiation of the program in 1996, JCAHO has changed the definition of a sentinel event to add more detail, instituted procedural revisions on reporting, authorized on-site review of root cause analyses to minimize risk of additional liability exposure, and altered the procedures for affecting a facility's accreditation status (and disclosing this change to the public) while an event is being investigated.[8] However, concerns remain regarding the confidentiality of data reported to JCAHO and the extent to which the information on a sentinel event is no longer protected under peer review if it is shared with JCAHO (these issues are discussed in Chapter 6).

There is the potential for cooperation between the JCAHO sentinel event program and state adverse event tracking programs. For example, JCAHO is currently working with New York State so that hospitals that report to the state's program are considered to be in compliance with JCAHO's sentinel events program.[9] This will reduce the need for hospitals to report to multiple groups with different requirements for each. The state and JCAHO are also seeking to improve communications between the two organizations before and after hospitals are surveyed for accreditation.

Medication Errors Reporting (MER) Program

The MER program is a voluntary medication error reporting system originated by the Institute for Safe Medication Practice (ISMP) in 1975 and administered today by U.S. Pharmacopeia (USP). The MER program receives reports from frontline practitioners via mail, telephone, or the Internet. Information is also shared with the FDA and the pharmaceutical companies mentioned in the reports. ISMP also publishes error reports received from USP in 16 publications every month and produces a biweekly publication and periodic special alerts that go to all hospitals in the United States. The MER program has received approximately 3,000 reports since 1993, primarily identifying new and emerging problems based on reports from people on the frontline.

MedMARx from the U.S. Pharmacopoeia

In August 1998, U.S. Pharmacopeia initiated the MedMARx program, an Internet-based, anonymous, voluntary system for hospitals to report medication errors. Hospitals subscribe to the program. Hospital employees may then report a medication error anonymously to MedMARx by completing a standardized report. Hospital management is then able to retrieve compiled data on its own facility and also obtain nonidentified comparative information on other participating hospitals. All information reported to MedMARx remains anonymous. All data and correspondence are tied to a confidential facility identification number. Information is not shared with FDA at this time. The JCAHO framework for conducting a root cause analysis is on the system for the convenience of reporters to download the forms, but the programs are not integrated.

Aviation Safety Reporting System at NASA

The three voluntary reporting systems described above represent focused initiatives that apply to a particular type of organization (e.g., hospital) or particular type of error (e.g., medication error). The Aviation Safety Reporting System (ASRS) is a voluntary, confidential incident reporting system used to identify hazards and latent system deficiencies in order to eliminate or mitigate them.[10] ASRS is described as an example of a comprehensive voluntary reporting system.

ASRS receives "incident" reports, defined as an occurrence associated with the operation of an aircraft that affects or could affect the safety of operations. Reports into ASRS are submitted by individuals confidentially. After any additional information is obtained through follow-up with reporters, the information is maintained anonymously in a database (reports submitted anonymously are not accepted). ASRS is designed to capture near misses, which are seen as fruitful areas for designing solutions to prevent future accidents.

The National Transportation Safety Board (NTSB) investigates aviation accidents. An "accident" is defined as an occurrence that results in death or serious injury or in which the aircraft receives substantial damage. NTSB was formed in 1967 and ASRS in 1976. The investigation of accidents thus preceded attention to near misses.

ASRS operates independently from the Federal Aviation Administration (FAA). It was originally formed under FAA, but operations were shifted to the National Aeronautics and Space Administration (NASA) because of the reluctance of pilots to report incidents (as differentiated from accidents) to a regulatory authority. FAA funds the ASRS, but NASA administers and manages the program independently. ASRS has no regulatory or enforcement powers over civil aviation.

ASRS issues alerts to the industry on hazards it identifies as needed (e.g., ASRS does not go through a regulatory agency to issue an alert or other communication; Linda Connell, Director of ASRS, personal communication, May 20, 1999). If a situation is very serious, it may issue an alert after only one incident. Often, ASRS has received multiple reports and noted a pattern. The purpose of ASRS alerts and other communications is to notify others of problems. Alerts may be disseminated throughout the industry and may also be communicated to the FAA to notify them about areas that may require action. ASRS does not propose or advocate specific solutions because it believes this would interfere with its role as an "honest broker" for reporters. As a result, although some reported problems may be acted upon, others are not. For example, ASRS has been notifying FAA and the industry about problems that have persisted throughout its 23-year history, such as problems with call signs. To date, no agency has been able to a find permanent solution. However, ASRS continues to issue alerts about the problem to remind people that the problem has not been solved.

ASRS maintains a database on reported incidents, identifies hazards and patterns in the data, conducts analyses on types of incidents, and interviews reporters when indicated. It sends out alert messages, publishes a monthly safety bulletin that is distributed to 85,000 readers and produces a semiannual safety topics publication targeted to the operators and flight crews of complex aircraft. Quick-response studies may be conducted for NTSB and FAA as needed (e.g., if an accident occurred, they may look for similar incidents). ASRS receives over 30,000 reports annually and has an operating budget of approximately $2 million.[11]

A more recent program is the Aviation Safety Action Programs. The de-identification of reports submitted to ASRS means that organizations do not have access to reports that identify problems in their own operations. In 1997, FAA established a demonstration program for the creation of Aviation Safety Action Programs (ASAP).[12] Under ASAP, an employee may submit a report on a serious incident that does not meet the threshold of an accident to the airline and the FAA with pilot and flight identification. Reports are reviewed at a regular meeting of an event review committee that includes representatives from the employee group, FAA and the airline. Corrective actions are identified as needed.

Mandatory Internal Reporting with Audit

Occupational Safety and Health Administration

OSHA uses a different approach for reporting than the systems already described. It requires companies to keep internal records of injury and illness, but does not require that the data be routinely submitted. The records must be made available during on-site inspections and may be required if the company is included in an annual survey of a sample of companies.[13] OSHA and the Bureau of Labor Statistics both conduct sample surveys and collect the routine data maintained by the companies. These agencies conduct surveys to construct incidence rates on worksite illness and injury that are tracked over time or to examine particular issues of concern, such as a certain activity.

Employers with 11 or more employees must routinely maintain records of occupational injury and illness as they occur. Employees have access to a summary log of the injury and illness reports, and to copies of any citations issued by OSHA. Citations must be posted for three days or until the problem is corrected, whichever is longer. Companies with ten or fewer employers are exempt from keeping such records unless they are selected for an annual survey and are required to report for that period. Some industries, although required to comply with OSHA rules, are not subject to record-keeping requirements (including some retail, trade, insurance, real estate, and services). However, they must still report the most serious accidents (defined as an accident that results in at least one death or five or more hospitalizations).

Key Points from Existing Reporting Systems

There are a number of ways that reporting systems can contribute to improving patient safety. Good reporting systems are a tool for gathering sufficient information about errors from multiple reporters to try to understand the factors that contribute to them and subsequently prevent their recurrence throughout the health care system. Feedback and dissemination of information can create an awareness of problems that have been encountered elsewhere and an expectation that errors should be fixed and safety is important. Finally, a larger-scale effort may improve analytic power by increasing the number of "rare" events reported. A serious error may not occur frequently enough in a single entity to be detected as a systematic problem; it is perceived as a random occurrence. On a larger scale, a trend may be easier to detect.

Reporting systems are particularly useful in their ability to detect unusual events or emerging problems.[14] Unusual events are easier to detect and report because they are rare, whereas common events are viewed as part of the "normal" course. For example, a poorly designed medical device that malfunctions routinely becomes viewed as a normal risk and one that practitioners typically find ways to work around. Some common errors may be recognized and reported, but many are not. Reporting systems also potentially allow for a fast response to a problem since reports come in spontaneously as an event occurs and can be reacted to quickly.

Two challenges that confront reporting systems are getting sufficient participation in the programs and building an adequate response system. All reporting programs, whether mandatory or voluntary, are perceived to suffer from underreporting. Indeed, some experts assert that all reporting is fundamentally voluntary since even mandated reporting can be avoided.[15] However, some mandatory programs receive many reports and some voluntary programs receive fewer reports. New York's mandatory program receives an average of 20,000 reports annually, while a leading voluntary program, the MER Program, has received approximately 3,000 reports since 1993. Reporting adverse reactions to medications to FDA is voluntary for practitioners, and they are not subject to FDA regulation (so the report is not going to an authority that can take action against them). Yet, underreporting is still perceived.[16] Of the approximately 235,000 reports received annually at FDA, 90 percent come from manufacturers (although practitioners may report to the manufacturers who report to FDA). Only about 10 percent are reported directly through MedWatch, mainly from practitioners.

The volume of reporting is influenced by more factors than simply whether reporting is mandatory or voluntary. Several reasons have been suggested for underreporting. One factor is related to confidentiality. As already described, many of the states contacted faced concerns about confidentiality, and what information should be released and when. Although patients were never identified, states varied on whether to release the identity of organizations. They were faced with having to balance the concerns of health care organizations to encourage participation in the program and the importance of making information available to protect and inform consumers. Voluntary programs often set up special procedures to protect the confidentiality of the information they receive. The issue of data protection and discoverability is discussed in greater detail in Chapter 6.

Another set of factors that affects the volume of reports relates to reporter perceptions and abilities. Feedback to reporters is believed to influence participation levels.[17] Belief by reporters that the information is actually used assures them that the time taken to file a report is worthwhile. Reporters need to perceive a benefit for reporting. This is true for all reporting systems, whether mandatory or voluntary. Health care organizations that are trained and educated in event recognition are also more likely to report events.[18] Clear standards, definitions, and tools are also believed to influence reporting levels. Clarity and ease helps reporters know what is expected to be reported and when. One experiment tried paying for reporting. This increased reporting while payments were provided, but the volume was not sustained after payments stopped.[19]

Although some reporting systems that focus on adverse events, such as hospital patients experiencing nosocomial infections, are used to develop incidence rates and track changes in these rates over time, caution must be exercised when calculating rates from adverse event reporting systems for several reasons. Many reporting systems are considered to be "passive" in that they rely on a report being submitted by someone who has observed the event.[20] "Active" systems work with participating health care organizations to collect complete data on an issue being tracked to determine rates of an adverse event[21] (e.g., the CDC conducted an active surveillance study of vaccine events with four HMOs linking vaccination records with hospital admission records[22]).

The low occurrence of serious errors can also produce wide variations in frequency from year to year. Some organizations and individuals may routinely report more than others, either because they are more safety conscious or because they have better internal systems.[23] Certain characteristics of medical processes may make it difficult to identify an adverse event, which can also lead to variation in reporting. For example, adverse drug events are difficult to detect when they are widely separated in time from the original use of the drug or when the reaction occurs commonly in an unexposed population.[24] These reasons make it difficult to develop reliable rates from reporting systems, although it may be possible to do so in selected cases. However, even without a rate, repetitive reports flag areas of concern that require attention.

It is important to note, however, that the goal of reporting programs is not to count the number of reports. The volume of reports by itself does not indicate the success of a program. Analyzing and using the information they provide and attaching the right tools, expertise and resources to the information contained in the reports helps to correct errors. Medication errors are heavily monitored, by several public and private reporting systems, some of which afford anonymous reporting. It is possible for a practitioner to voluntarily and confidentially report a medication error to the FDA or to private systems (e.g., MER program, MedMARx). Some states with mandatory reporting may also receive reports of medication-related adverse events. Yet, some medication problems continue to occur, such as unexpected deaths from the availability of concentrated potassium chloride on patient care units.[25]

Reporting systems without adequate resources for analysis and follow-up action are not useful. Reporting without analysis or follow-up may even be counterproductive in that it weakens support for constructive responses and is viewed as a waste of resources. Although exact figures are not available, it is generally believed that the analysis of reports is harder to do, takes longer and costs more than data collection. Being able to conduct good analyses also requires that the information received through reporting systems is adequate. People involved in the operation of reporting systems believe it is better to have good information on fewer cases than poor information on many cases. The perceived value of reports (in any type of reporting system) lies in the narrative that describes the event and the circumstances under which it occurred. Inadequate information provides no benefit to the reporter or the health system.

DISCUSSION OF COMMITTEE RECOMMENDATIONS

Reporting systems may have a primary focus on accountability or on safety improvement. Design features vary depending on the primary purpose. Accountability systems are mandatory and usually receive reports on errors that resulted in serious harm or death; safety improvement systems are generally voluntary and often receive reports on events resulting in less serious harm or no harm at all. Accountability systems tend to receive reports from organizations; safety improvement systems may receive reports from organizations or frontline practitioners. Accountability systems may release information to the public; safety improvement systems are more likely to be confidential.

Figure 5.1 presents a proposed hierarchy of reporting, sorting potential errors into two categories: (1) errors that result in serious injury or death (i.e., serious preventable adverse events), and (2) lesser injuries or noninjurious events (near-misses).[26] Few errors cause serious harm or death; that is the tip of the triangle. Most errors result in less or no harm, but may represent early warning signs of a system failure with the potential to cause serious harm or death.

The committee believes that the focus of mandatory reporting systems should be on the top tier of the triangle in Figure 5.1. Errors in the lower tier are issues that might be the focus of voluntary external reporting systems, as well as research projects supported by the Center for Patient Safety and internal patient safety programs of health care organizations. The core reporting formats and measures promulgated by the National Forum for Health Care Quality Measurement and Reporting should focus first on the top tier. Additional standardized formats and measures pertaining to other

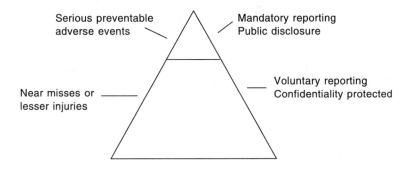

FIGURE 5-1 Hierarchy of reporting.

types of errors might be promulgated in the future to serve as tools to be made available to voluntary reporting systems or health care organizations for quality improvement purposes.

The committee believes there is an important role for both mandatory and voluntary reporting systems. Mandatory reporting of serious adverse events is essential for public accountability and the current practices are too lax, both in enforcement of the requirements for reporting and in the regulatory responses to these reports. The public has the right to expect health care organizations to respond to evidence of safety hazards by taking whatever steps are necessary to make it difficult or impossible for a similar event to occur in the future. The public also has the right to be informed about unsafe conditions. Requests by providers for confidentiality and protection from liability seem inappropriate in this context. At the same time, the committee recognizes that appropriately designed voluntary reporting systems have the potential to yield information that will impact significantly on patient safety and can be widely disseminated. The reports and analyses in these reporting systems should be protected from disclosure for legal liability purposes.

Mandatory Reporting of Serious Adverse Events

The committee believes there should be a mandatory reporting program for serious adverse events, implemented nationwide, linked to systems of accountability, and made available to the public. Comparable to aviation "accidents" that are investigated by the National Transportation Safety Board, health care organizations should be required to submit reports on the most serious adverse events using a standard format. The types of adverse events to be reported may include, for example, maternal deaths; deaths or serious injuries associated with the use of a new device, operation or medication; deaths following elective surgery or anesthetic deaths in Class I patients. In light of the sizable number of states that have already established mandatory reporting systems, the committee thinks it would be wise to build on this experience in creating a standardized reporting system that is implemented nationwide.

Within these objectives, however, there should be flexibility in implementation. Flexibility and innovation are important in this stage of development because the existing state programs have used different approaches to implement their programs and a "best practice" or preferred approach is not yet known. The Center for Patient Safety can support states in identifying and communicating best practices. States could choose to collect and analyze such data themselves. Alternatively, they could rely on an accrediting body, such as Joint Commission for Accreditation of Healthcare Organizations or the National Committee for Quality Assurance, to perform the function for them as many states do now for licensing surveys. States could also contract with peer review organizations (PROs) to perform the function. As noted in Chapter 4, the Center for Patient Safety should evaluate the approaches taken by states in implementing reporting programs. States have employed a variety of strategies in their programs, yet few (if any) have been subject to rigorous evaluation. Program features that might be evaluated include: factors that encourage or inhibit reporting, methods of analyzing reports, roles and responsibilities of health care organizations and the state in investigating adverse events, follow-up actions taken by states, information disclosed to the public, and uses of the information by consumers and purchasers.

Although states should have flexibility in how they choose to implement the reporting program, all state programs should require reporting for a standardized core set of adverse events that result in death or serious injury, and the information reported should also be standardized.

The committee believes that these standardized reporting formats should be developed by an organization with the following characteristics. First, it should be a public–private partnership, to reflect the need for involvement by both sectors and the potential use of the reporting format by both the public and the private sectors. Second, it should be broadly representative, to reflect the input from many different stakeholders that have an interest in patient safety. Third, it should be able to gather the expertise needed for the task. This requires adequate financial resources, as well as sufficient standing to involve the leading experts. Enabling legislation can support all three objectives.

The National Forum for Health Care Quality Measurement and Reporting meets these criteria. The purpose of this public-private partnership (formed in May 1999) is to develop a comprehensive quality measurement and public reporting strategy that addresses priorities for quality measurement for all stakeholders consistent with national aims for quality improvement in health care. It is to develop a plan for implementing quality measurement, data collection and reporting standards; identify core sets of measures; and promote standardized measurement specifications. One of its specific tasks should relate to patient safety.

The advantage of using the Forum is that its goal already is to develop a

measurement framework for quality generally. A focus on safety would ensure that safety gets built into a broader quality agenda. A public–private
partnership would also be able to convene the mix of stakeholders who, it is
hoped, would subsequently adopt the standards and standardized reporting
recommendations of the Forum. However, the Forum is a new organization
that is just starting to come together; undoubtedly some time will be required to build the organization and set its agenda.

Federal enabling legislation and support will be required to direct the
National Forum for Health Care Quality Measurement and Reporting to
promulgate standardized reporting requirements for serious adverse events
and encourage all states to implement the minimum reporting requirements.
Such federal legislation pertaining to state roles may be modeled after the
Health Insurance Portability and Accountability Act of 1996 (HIPAA).
HIPAA provides three options for implementing a program: (1) states may
pass laws congruent with or stronger than the federal floor and enforce them
using state agencies; (2) they may create an acceptable alternative mechanism and enforce it with state agencies; or finally, (3) they may decline to
pass new laws or modify existing ones and leave enforcement of HIPAA to
the federal government.[27] OSHA is similarly designed in that states may
develop their own OSHA program with matching funds from the federal
government; the federal OSHA program is employed in states that have not
formed a state-level program.

Voluntary Reporting Systems

The committee believes that voluntary reporting systems play a valuable
role in encouraging improvements in patient safety and are a complement to
mandatory reporting systems. The committee considered whether a national
voluntary reporting system should be established similar to the Aviation
Safety Reporting System. Compared to mandatory reporting, voluntary reporting systems usually receive reports from frontline practitioners who can
report hazardous conditions that may or may not have resulted in patient
harm. The aim is to learn about these potential precursors to errors and try
to prevent a tragedy from occurring.

The committee does not propose a national voluntary reporting system
for several reasons. First, there are already a number of good efforts, particularly in the area of medications. Three complementary national reporting systems are focused on medication errors: FDA, the Institute for Safe
Medication Practice, and U.S. Pharmacopeia. The JCAHO sentinel events

program is another existing national reporting program for hospitals that will also receive reports on medication and other errors. These reporting systems should be encouraged and promoted within health care organizations, and better use should be made of available information being reported to them.

Second, there are several options available about how to design such a voluntary reporting system. Better information is needed on what would be the best approach. At least three different approaches were identified. One is a universal, voluntary reporting system, modeled after ASRS. The concern with this approach is the potential volume of reports that might come forward when such a system is applied to health care. Another concern is that any single group is unlikely to have the expertise needed to analyze and interpret the diverse set of issues raised in health care. The experience of ASRS has shown that the analysts reviewing incoming reports must be content experts who can understand and interpret these reports.[28] In health care, different expertise is likely needed to analyze, for example, medication errors, equipment problems, problems in the intensive care unit (ICU), pediatric problems, and home care problems.

Another approach is to develop focused "mini-systems" that are targeted toward selected areas (e.g., those that exist for medications) rather than a single voluntary program. This approach would manage the potential volume of reports and match the expertise to the problems. It is possible that there should be different mini-systems for different issues such as medications, surgery, pediatrics, and so forth. If such mini-systems are formed, there should be a mechanism for sharing information across them since a report to one system may have relevance for another (e.g., surgical events that also involve medications).

A third possibility is to use a sampling approach. For example, in its postmarketing surveillance of medical devices, FDA is moving away from a universal reporting system for hospitals and nursing homes to one in which a representative sample of hospitals and nursing homes keeps complete data. Its pilot test found that both the quantity and the quality of reports improved when FDA worked with a sample of hospitals who were trained in error identification and reporting and could receive feedback quickly. By periodically renewing the sample, the burden on any organization is limited (although participation in the sample may have the side benefit of helping interested organizations build their internal systems and train practitioners in error detection).

Lastly, establishing a comprehensive voluntary reporting system modeled after ASRS would require an enormous investment of time and resources. The committee believes that recommending such an investment would be premature in light of the many questions still surrounding this issue.

The committee does believe that voluntary reporting systems have a very important role to play in enhancing understanding of the factors that contribute to errors. When properly structured, voluntary systems can help to keep participating health care organizations focused on patient safety issues through frequent communication about emerging concerns and potential safety improvement strategies. Voluntary systems can provide much-needed expertise and information to health care organizations and providers.

The continued development of voluntary reporting efforts should be encouraged. Through its various outreach activities, the Center for Patient Safety should describe and disseminate information on voluntary reporting programs throughout the health care industry and should periodically convene sponsors and users of voluntary reporting systems to discuss ways in which these systems can be made more effective. As a part of developing the national research agenda for safety, the Center for Patient Safety should consider projects that might lead to the development of knowledge and tools that would enhance the effectiveness of voluntary reporting programs. The Center should also periodically assess whether there are gaps in the current complement of voluntary reporting programs and should consider funding pilot projects.

In summary, this chapter and the previous chapter outlining the proposed Center for Patient Safety together describe a comprehensive approach for improving the availability of information about medical errors and using the information to design systems that are safer for patients. Although this chapter focuses on using reporting systems to learn about and learn from errors that have already occurred, Chapter 4 focused on how to create and disseminate new knowledge for building safer delivery systems. Both of these strategies should work together to make health care safer for patients.

REFERENCES

1. Bates, David, W.; Spell, Nathan; Cullen, David J., et al. The Costs of Adverse Drug Events in Hospitalized Patients. *JAMA*. 277(4):307–311, 1997.

2. For example, there are several efforts relative to the reporting of medication errors specifically, such as the Institute for Safe Medication Practices (ISMP) and U.S. Pharmacopeia. The FDA sponsors its MedWatch medication and device reporting program. The National Coordinating Council of the Medical Errors Program (NCC-MERP)

has developed a taxonomy for medication errors for the recording and tracking of errors. General reporting programs (not specific to medications) include JCAHO's sentinel events reporting program and some state programs.

3. "State Agency Experiences Regarding Mandatory Reporting of Sentinel Events," JCAHO draft survey results, April 1999.

4. Billings, Charles, "Incident Reporting Systems in Medicine and Experience With the Aviation Safety Reporting System," in Cook, Richard; Woods, David; and Miller, Charlotte, *A Tale of Two Stories: Contrasting Views of Patient Safety*, Chicago: National Patient Safety Foundation of the AMA, 1998.

5. Office of the Inspector General, "The External Review of Hospital Quality: A Call for Greater Accountability," http://www.dhhs.gov/progorg/oei/reports/oei-01-97-00050.htm.

6. Additional strategies include field investigations, epidemiological studies and other focused studies.

7. "Sentinel Event Policy and Procedure," Revised: July 18, 1998. Joint Commission on Accreditation of Healthcare Organizations, Oakbrook Terrace, Illinois.

8. Joint Commission on Accreditation of Healthcare Organizations, Sentinel Event Alert, Number Three, May 1, 1998.

9. Heigel, Fred, presentation at 12th Annual State Health Policy Conference, National Academy for State Health Policy, Cincinnati, Ohio, August 2, 1999.

10. "Federal Aviation Administration, Office of System Safety, Safety Data," http://nasdac.faa.gov/safety_data.

11. Billings, Charles, "Incident Reporting Systems in Medicine and Experience With the Aviation Safety Reporting System," Appendix B in *A Tale of Two Stories*, Richard Cook, David Woods and Charlotte Miller, Chicago: National Health Care Safety Council of the National Patient Safety Foundation at the AMA, 1998.

12. Federal Aviation Administration, "Aviation Safety Action Programs (ASAP)," Advisory Circular No. 120-66, 1/8/97.

13. "All About OSHA," U.S. Department of Labor, Occupational Safety and Health Administration, OSHA 2056, 1995 (Revised).

14. Brewer, Timothy and Colditz, Graham A. Postmarketing Surveillance and Adverse Drug Reactions, Current Perspectives and Future Needs. *JAMA*. 281(9):824-829, 1999. See also: FDA, "Managing the Risks from Medical Product Use, Creating a Risk Management Framework," Report to the FDA Commissioner from the Task Force on Risk Management, USDHHS, May, 1999.

15. Billings, Charles, presentation to Subcommittee on Creating an External Environment for Quality Health Care, January 29, 1999.

16. Brewer and Colditz, 1999. See also: FDA, "Managing the Risks from Medical Product Use," May 1999.

17. FDA, "Managing the Risks from Medical Product Use," May 1999.

18. As part of the FDA Modernization Act of 1997, the FDA is mandated to shift from a universal mandatory reporting system for users (hospitals and nursing homes) of medical devices to one where only a subset of facilities report. In their pilot test, they believed that faster and better feedback to reporters contributed to improved reporting. FDA, May 1999. See also: Susan Gardner, Center for Devices and Radiological Health, personal communication, November 24, 1998.

19. Feely, John; Moriarty, Siobhan; O'Connor, Patricia. Stimulating Reporting of Adverse Drug Reactions by Using a Fee. *BMJ*. 300:22–23, 1990.

20. FDA, "Managing the Risks from Medical Product Use," 1999.

21. Brewer and Colditz, 1999.

22. Farrington, Paddy; Pugh, Simon; Colville, Alaric, et al. A New Method for Active Surveillance of Adverse Events from Diphtheria/Tetanus/Pertussis and Measles/Mumps/Rubella Vaccines. *Lancet*. 345(8949):567–569, 1995.

23. Nagel, David C., "Human Error In Aviation Operations," in D.C. Nagel and E.L. Wiener (eds.), *Human Factors in Aviation*, eds., Orlando, FL: Academic Press, Inc., 1988.

24. Brewer and Colditz, 1999.

25. Medication Error Prevention—Potassium Chloride. *JCAHO Sentinel Event Alert*, Issue One, Oakbrook Terrace, Illinois: 1998.

26. Adapted from work by JCAHO based on presentation by Margaret VanAmringe to the Subcommittee on Creating an External Environment for Quality in Health Care, June 15, 1999, Washington, D.C.

27. Nichols, Len M. and Blumberg, Linda J. A Different Kind of "New Federalism"? The Health Insurance Portability and Accountability Act of 1996. *Health Affairs*. 17(3):25–42, 1998.

28. Billings, Charles, presentation to Subcommittee on Creating an External Environment for Quality, January 29, 1999.

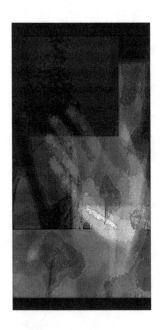

6
Protecting Voluntary Reporting Systems from Legal Discovery

Although all industries face concerns about liability, the organization of health care creates a different set of circumstances compared to other industries. In health care, physicians primarily determine the amount and content of care rendered. A hospital or clinic often produces the care directed by the physician. The consumer, purchaser, and health plan share in decisions to determine whether and how treatment decisions directed by the physician are paid, which influences access to care. Although some of these decisions could be under one umbrella, they are often dispersed across different and unrelated entities. Compared to other industries, there is no single responsible entity in health care that is held accountable for an episode of care. The physician, in particular, has a significant responsibility for the well-being of his or her patients and the decisions made concerning their care. This distinctive arrangement in organization and decision making in health care creates a unique set of liability issues and challenges in creating an environment conducive to recognizing and learning from errors.

The potential for litigation may sometimes significantly influence the behavior of physicians and other health care providers. Often the interests of the various participants in furnishing an episode of care are not aligned and may be antagonistic to each other. In this environment, physicians and other providers can be cautious about providing information that may be subsequently used against them. Thus, the prominence of litigation can be a substantial deterrent to the development and maintenance of the reporting systems discussed in this report.

Chapter 5 lays out a strategy to encourage greater recognition and analysis of errors and improvements in patient safety through a mandatory reporting system for errors that result in serious harm, and voluntary participation in error reporting systems that focus on "near misses" or errors resulting in lesser harm. The issue of whether data submitted to reporting systems should be protected from disclosure, particularly in litigation, arose early in the committee discussions. Members of the committee had different views. Some believed all information should be protected because access to the information by outsiders created concerns with potential litigation and interfered with disclosure of errors and taking actions to improve safety. Others believed that information should be disclosed because the public has a right to know. Liability is part of the system of accountability and serves a legitimate role in holding people responsible for their actions.

The recommendations contained in Chapter 5 and in this chapter reflect the committee's recognition of the legitimacy of the alternative views. The committee believes that errors that are identified through a mandatory reporting system and are part of a public system of accountability should not be protected from discovery. Other events that are reported inside health care organizations or to voluntary systems should be protected because they often focus on lesser injuries or non-injurious events that have the potential to cause serious harm to patients, but have not produced a serious adverse event that requires reporting to the mandatory system. Protecting such information encourages disclosure of problems and a proactive approach to correcting problems before serious harm occurs.

Although information about serious injuries and deaths due to errors should not be protected from discovery, it is important that information released to the public is accurate. As described in Chapter 5, mandatory reporting systems receive reports on adverse events, which are then investigated to determine whether an error occurred. The mere filing of a report should not, by itself, trigger release of information. Rather, information should be released after an investigation has been completed so the information that is released is accurate. This chapter focuses primarily on protecting information reported to voluntary systems, although aspects may also apply to protecting data submitted to mandatory systems until the information is ready for public release.

The committee believes that a different approach to promoting the collection, sharing, and analysis of such data (not considered in this chapter) would be to change the legal environment in which health care organizations and providers operate. Exclusive enterprise liability, shifting liability for medical injuries from individual practitioners to responsible organizations, has been suggested to possess several advantages over the current liability system.[1-3] One of these is to remove the fear of personal liability from individual health care workers, eliminating this incentive to hide errors. Another proposed reform, no-fault compensation for medical injuries, might promote reporting by eliminating the adversarial inquiry into fault and blame that characterizes the current liability system.[4] Workplace injuries to employees are handled within an example of such a no-fault, enterprise-liability system.[5]

Together, enterprise liability and no-fault compensation might produce a legal environment more conducive to reporting and analysis, without the elaborate legal and practical strategies needed to protect data under the current liability system. An analysis of enterprise liability and no-fault compensation systems is beyond the scope of the Quality of Health Care in America project, but the committee believes that the issue merits further analysis.

This chapter examines legal precedents and practical experiences bearing on how and to what extent information can be protected in error reporting systems when it leaves the health care organization that generated it. Legal protections like state peer review shields and laws created to protect a specific reporting system have much promise. Many current state peer review statutes, however, may not protect data about errors shared in collaborative networks, especially across state lines, or reported to voluntary reporting systems (e.g., independent data banks). A combination of practical and legal safeguards may be the best approach to protect the data in voluntary reporting systems from discoverability. The practical safeguards of anonymous reporting and de-identification (removal of identifying information after receipt of the report) can confer some, but not complete, protection. Statutory protection could add three benefits to some level of de-identification: (1) it could provide an added measure of security for the data; (2) it could protect from subpoena identifiable reporters and recipients of the reports; and (3) it could permit the reporting system to obtain and retain information that might identify the reports and reporters.

RECOMMENDATION

RECOMMENDATION 6.1 Congress should pass legislation to extend peer review protections to data related to patient safety and quality improvement that are collected and analyzed by health care organizations for internal use or shared with others solely for purposes of improving safety and quality.

Existing law often shields data about errors within an institution, but this protection may be lost when the data are transmitted elsewhere, for example, to other institutions collaborating in an error reduction initiative or to a voluntary reporting system. Unless such data are assured protection, people will be reluctant to discuss them and opportunities to improve will be lost. A more conducive legal environment is needed to encourage health care professionals and organizations to identify, analyze, and prevent errors without increasing the threat of litigation and without compromising patients' legal rights. Information about errors which have resulted in serious harm or death to patients and which are subject to mandatory reporting should not be protected.

INTRODUCTION

The systematic reporting and tracking of safety problems is an important approach to quality improvement. There are many ways to gather, maintain, and use safety-related data. Systems can vary considerably according to their key characteristics (e.g., type of events reported, who reports, voluntary or mandatory submission, location and maintenance of a data bank), which also affect the likelihood of vulnerability to discovery in legal process.

All such systems face two bedrock issues: (1) how to motivate health care practitioners and others to submit information, and (2) how to maintain reported data in a systematic way that is useful to practitioners. A central concern for both is the extent to which confidentiality of information should be maintained given a litigious society. Access to detailed information compiled by peer reviewers, risk managers, or others could greatly help a plaintiff's lawyer to build and prove a case. This in turn creates a strong disincentive to collect and report such information.

Plaintiffs' interest in and uses of information on errors depend on the level of identification of the data. A fully identified report will always be of interest to the plaintiff involved in the case reported. But even if the data are identified or aggregated by institution or physician, but not by patient, they may still be useful in claims against the institution for negligent supervision or credentialing—causes of action that are well known to the plaintiff's bar. Data from which all personal and organizational identifiers have been removed could still be used to prove some elements of certain types of cases, such as causation (e.g., injuries similar to the plaintiff's were caused by the same mechanism or problem; there was reason for the defendant to know of problems with a certain process or device). The latter use is probably not common today, possibly in part because of the scarcity of such data. The more that liability moves from individual focus to a focus on organizations, the more useful general information may become.

Plaintiffs can seek information from three components of a reporting system: (1) the original reporter; (2) the personnel who receive, investigate, or analyze the reports; and (3) the data per se as they reside in the data bank. The way in which plaintiffs can gain access to these targets is described in the next section. Two avenues are available to protect each of these targets: laws that prevent discovery and practical methods that render the reporter unfindable or the data unuseful to the plaintiff. These protections may apply differently to the three possible targets of discovery. They are described in more detail, along with the experience that reporting systems have had with them. The purpose of the analysis is to illuminate the legal policy and design choices facing those who want to protect data collection, sharing, and analysis of information on adverse events and errors.

The committee notes that protecting data in a reporting system as recommended in this chapter does not mean that the plaintiff in a lawsuit could not try to obtain such information through other avenues if it is important in securing redress for harm; it just means that the plaintiff would not be assisted by the presence of a reporting system designed specifically for other purposes beneficial to society.

THE BASIC LAW OF EVIDENCE AND DISCOVERABILITY OF ERROR-RELATED INFORMATION

Demands for information on errors can come from any of the plaintiffs in medical malpractice lawsuits, which are almost always based on state law.* Whether and when plaintiffs can obtain access to such data or have such information admitted as evidence at trial depend on the general rules of evidence and civil procedure, as applied by a state judge under particular

---

*Error data may be sought in other types of cases as well, such as antitrust or libel claims by physicians against medical organizations. Further, regulators may seek data on injuries, either under their general authority (notably, state licensing boards that can discipline practitioners) or under specific statutory schemes of regulation that mandate reporting and investigation of consequential errors (discussed below).

circumstances. Rules vary by state, but most are similar to the federal rules described below. State differences are mentioned when relevant.

Trial Admissibility and the Rule of Relevance

The basic legal principle governing whether information can be used by a plaintiff in a civil trial is the rule of relevance. The formal threshold of relevance is quite low: whether the evidence would have "any tendency" to make any element of the cause of action (mainly, existence of negligence, causation of harm, presence of damages) more or less likely.[6] Moreover, trial judges are accorded broad discretion in judging whether an item of evidence is relevant,[7] and they make such determinations on a case-by-case basis.[8] In practice, then, a piece of evidence is relevant to a particular case if the judge says it is, unless there is no arguable basis for its relevance.

All relevant evidence is admissible at trial unless there is a specific exception or reason for it to be inadmissible,[9] such as the evidentiary privileges discussed below. The attorney–client privilege, for example, can prevent certain clearly relevant statements by the client from being introduced at trial.

Information on errors could be relevant to a malpractice lawsuit in three ways. First, if the data are reported about the *particular case in dispute*, so that the report and the litigation are about the identical circumstances, every piece of information would undoubtedly be relevant. This use of data would apply only to databases with identified data about errors that produce injury; the specific identification is what makes the information relevant, and the data would help establish liability in the lawsuit. The information could show negligence, causation (i.e., relation of the injury to the medical care that prompted the report), and possible damages.

Second, information about *similar occurrences* to the case in dispute is relevant to lawsuits that allege not merely one negligent occurrence, but negligence in a practitioners' engaging in a certain activity at all. It may be argued that an individual doctor's record makes it negligent to fail to refer a patient to a better-qualified practitioner. Similarly, a suit may allege negligent oversight in credentialing or supervision by the institution, medical group or health plan within which the doctor practices. In such a lawsuit, the plaintiff would argue that the occurrence of similar problems before the case in dispute should have or did put the defendant on notice of a pattern of problems that should have been corrected before the plaintiff's injury occurred. The previous occurrences would have to be similar in salient aspects to the data sought from the bank, for example, a particular sort of complex surgery. This use of prior similar-occurrence data would require data identified at least by institution, because the notice has to be shown with respect to a particular defendant. In one case, for example, a plaintiff who was injured by implantation of a pacemaker was allowed access to records of other instances of pacemaker implantation to help make a case for negligent supervision of the physicians by the hospital.[10]

Third, data on *similar occurrences* might also be relevant in more limited ways—to help some lawsuits prove certain aspects of their cases. If, for example, there is a dispute about whether a particular instrumentality could have caused the injury ("causation"), evidence that it caused similar injuries in other instances could be relevant. Other points that could be proven with similar-occurrence data include the defendant's ability to correct a known defect (e.g., a systems weakness or device problem), the lack of safety for intended uses, and the standard of care. Using similar occurrences in this manner would not require identified data, and the similar instances could have come before or after the event that is the subject of the lawsuit.

A recent Florida case combined the notice and causation purposes of similar-occurrence evidence. An obese patient alleged that the defendant obstetrician injured her child by delivering her on a standard bed, rather than a drop-down bed. The court held that the records of other obese patients the doctor had delivered were relevant and discoverable. If other infants suffered similar injuries when a standard bed was used, this should have afforded the obstetrician notice that this method was deficient. Conversely, if no such injuries occurred when drop-down beds were used, this might be relevant for causation. In this instance, the other patients' names were removed from the records.[11] A similar rationale could easily apply to a collection of data on errors.

Pretrial Discoverability

The potential for discovery is even greater than indicated by the preceding section on trial admissibility. The requirement of relevance applies to whether a piece of evidence can be admitted into the record at trial. A pretrial process called "discovery" can extend a plaintiff's reach even further by allowing the plaintiff access to information that would not be admissible at the trial, but could *lead* to admissible evidence at the subsequent trial. Discovery is the process by which each party can obtain evidence in the possession of the other party and nonparties. It typically consists of requests for copies of documents and questions asked under oath of the other party (called interrogatories if written and depositions if oral). It may also extend to the production of physical objects or even the plaintiff's person for a medical examination. Persons or organizations that are not parties in a lawsuit can also be compelled to provide verbal, documentary, or physical evidence.

Relevance for discovery purposes is broadly and liberally construed. If there is a doubt about relevance, judges will generally permit discovery.[12] The information asked for need not be admissible at trial, as long as it reasonably might lead to the discovery of admissible evidence.[13] Therefore, a report of a medical error need not itself be admissible to be discoverable. The report could point the plaintiff toward relevant facts needed to prove the case. The report could inform the plaintiff, for example, of theories or conclusions about what contributed to the occurrence of the error. This knowledge could help direct the plaintiff's search for admissible evidence, for example, by suggesting the existence or importance of pertinent documents, witnesses, and questions that the plaintiff would not have otherwise considered.

Nonparties

Discovery can be obtained from nonparties as well as parties to the action. Nonparties include any person or organization that is not named in the lawsuit as being allegedly liable for the injury. They could include external data banks, quality consultants, accrediting bodies such as JCAHO, and other persons or organizations that have information on errors. Subject to the judge's approval, the party seeking discovery simply issues a subpoena to the nonparty for the information.[14] The same methods of discovery generally apply to nonparties as to parties, except that interrogatories (a set of written questions) normally cannot be used with nonparties. With regard to the scope of discovery, the major difference for nonparties is that, if compliance with the subpoena would impose a burden on the nonparty, the court may impose a higher standard of relevance on the request for discovery. Judges may also be more apt to limit the scope or duration of a party's probing of a nonparty's information.

Judges are given substantial discretion over discovery from nonparties as well as discovery from parties to the lawsuit. Thus, the person or entity that reported or shared the error information, independent investigators, organizations that maintain information on errors, and those who work for such organizations could be subject to subpoenas, as long as compliance with the subpoena would not impose an undue burden. Even a data bank that maintains information with no personal or organizational identifiers would not protect a reporter to the data bank from being compelled to testify under oath about his or her recollections of the case, if the reporter could be identified by the plaintiff. The ease of identifying the reporter in practice is variable. It could be straightforward, for example, if a single physician was responsible for all quality assurance reviews in a medical group. Similarly, those who receive, de-identify, investigate, and analyze reports could be compelled to testify if they could be identified with sufficient particularity to be served with a subpoena.

LEGAL PROTECTIONS AGAINST DISCOVERY OF INFORMATION ABOUT ERRORS

Three main types of legal protections can block the discovery of data on errors. These include (1) general rules of evidence (not restricted to the medical context), (2) the medical peer review privilege, and (3) special statutory privileges enacted for particular reporting systems. This section discusses each of the protections in turn, along with their limitations.

General Rules of Evidence

Three general rules of evidence could potentially protect error information from disclosure—the remedial action privilege, the attorney–client privilege, and the work product doctrine. Each has some applicability to reporting systems, but each also has significant limits.

Remedial Action

By a long-standing rule of evidence, a showing that remedial action has been taken after an injury cannot be admitted as proof that the injury resulted from negligence or a defective product. One rationale for this rule is to encourage defendants and potential defendants to improve safety, without having to worry that doing so might be taken as an admission of prior substandard practice. The other rationale for the rule is that remedial measures are not necessarily relevant to negligence: that is, one can seek to prevent nonnegligent as well as negligent injuries. All states but one have adopted this rule.[15]

Some states have extended this rule to include self-evaluative reports or other postinjury analyses and reports. This might include evaluative reports on health care errors. The policy rationale for the rule would argue for this extension; without it, defendants might be unwilling to undertake the analyses needed to devise remedial measures. A California court, for example, recently held that the rule protected the records of peer review committees from discovery, independently from California's peer review statute, which also applied.[16]

However, other states have ruled the opposite way or have not yet reached the question of whether evaluative reports are protected.[17] Even in states that have extended the remedial measures rule to evaluative reports, protecting the reports outside of the institution involved in the lawsuit would require yet another extension of the rule. Another problem is that even if the reports are protected from being used by a plaintiff to prove the main elements of the cause of action (such as negligence), they could still be admissible for other purposes. A plaintiff could use them, for example, to impeach a witness (i.e., contradict a witness' testimony), prove causation, or prove the feasibility of taking preventive measures.[18]

Furthermore, the discovery privilege applies to critical evaluation (analysis, opinions, and conclusions) but not to facts of the event, so plaintiffs can still obtain factual information contained in the reports to support their case (e.g., what happened, who was there, what was said, whether the equipment was functioning normally).[19]

Attorney–Client Privilege

Communications with one's attorney are privileged from discovery. The purpose of the privilege is to encourage free communication between clients and lawyers so that clients may have the full benefit of legal advice. The privilege is nearly absolute, in that an opposing party can almost never argue that it should not be applied in particular circumstances.* It can be waived, however, by the client to whom it belongs; the attorney has a permanent obligation to the client and can never waive the privilege.

Attorney–client privilege will rarely if ever be useful in protecting reports sent to an external entity. Typically, the client is the medical institution,

---

*There are limited exceptions not relevant here, such as the duty of a lawyer as an officer of the court to report a client's plans to engage in future criminal activity.

which generally includes only senior management for purposes of this privilege. A report from a floor or charge nurse, for example, may not qualify. The most important problem, however, is that even if a document is originally covered by the attorney–client privilege, once it is sent to any nonparty, including external data banks or independent collaborating institutions, it loses the protection of the privilege. In other words, sending a report to one's attorney does not immunize it from discovery if it is also used for other purposes.

Attorney Work Product Doctrine

This rule protects materials that are created by or on behalf of a lawyer in preparation for litigation. The purpose is to protect the thoughts and plans of the lawyer, and the privilege can be waived only by the lawyer. Some states do not apply this doctrine to protect reports on errors, not even those kept internal to an organization, such as incident reports.[20] These states view the reports as being generated in the ordinary course of business. In addition, the protection afforded by the work product doctrine is not absolute; it can be overcome if the other party has need of the materials and would be unable without hardship to obtain the equivalent information.[21] In this situation, the facts of the event can be discovered, but the thoughts, opinions, and plans of the lawyer remain protected (i.e., may be removed before the materials are produced in discovery).

Peer Review Privilege

The peer review privilege is the most promising existing source of legal protection for data on errors. This privilege is statutory and is specific to medical peer review within specified settings and meeting specified standards. Every state, except one, statutorily protect from discovery various records and deliberations of peer review committees.*[22,23] The quality improvement purpose of peer review is consistent with the purpose of reporting systems; the statutes' value in protecting reporting, however, depends on fitting the reporting system to the specifics of each protective statute.

---

*New Jersey is the exception, according to a 50-state survey of peer review statutes that was undertaken in part to understand how JCAHO's proposed "sentinel event" reporting would fare under the statutes.

These statutes vary considerably in their reach and strength. Overall, this makes them a problematic source of legal protection for data on errors. Some protect only documents generated by the peer review committee, whereas others protect information provided to them. In addition, the treatment of incident reports within an institution, such as a hospital, varies by state. Some statutes have specific requirements for the composition of qualifying peer review committees (e.g., that physicians constitute a majority of the members). In some states, a hospital committee must be under the aegis of the medical staff, not the administrative staff.[24]

Some states restrict the privilege to in-hospital committees or committees of professional societies. Many statutes may not cover collaborations among institutions, even if all are within an integrated delivery system. The California statute is one of the broadest and might apply to collaborative reporting systems and external data banks. California defines a peer review body as including "a medical or professional staff of any licensed health care facility, a nonprofit medical professional society, or a committee whose function is to review the quality of professional care provided by the members or employees of the entity to which the committee belongs."[25] No statute expressly covers systems or collaborations that cross state lines.

States can develop statutes to accommodate reporting systems, such as in Oklahoma. In that state the law protects any information, including interviews, reports, statements, memoranda, or other data, that is provided "for use in the course of studies for the purpose of reducing morbidity or mortality." The recipients may use such information "only for the purpose of advancing medical research or medical education in the interest of reducing morbidity or mortality." The findings and conclusions resulting from these studies are also protected. The Oklahoma Supreme Court has upheld the protection under this statute for records generated by a hospital infectious disease committee that reviewed every case involving infection in order to improve infection control.[26] It would appear possible to devise reporting systems that would meet the requirements of this statute.

Even when peer review information qualifies for the privilege, it may nonetheless be discoverable under some circumstances. The information may not be protected in allegations of negligent supervision or credentialing by an institution, because the performance of the peer review process is what is at issue in such claims. Some state medical licensing boards have gained access to peer review information for disciplinary purposes.[27] Some state courts employ a balancing test to determine whether a plaintiff should have access to facts contained in peer review documents (though not opinions or conclusions), balancing how crucial this is to the plaintiff (e.g., not available in any other way) against how much trouble and expense it imposes on the defendant.* Moreover, state or federal law enforcement authorities may be able to discover the information for use in criminal proceedings, although instances of criminal prosecution for medical errors are exceptionally rare. Many states' statutes prevent a plaintiff from compelling a member of the peer review committee to testify, but one might testify voluntarily.[28] To close this loophole, hospitals can adopt bylaws prohibiting staff members from disclosing any information obtained through the peer review committee.

There is federal protection for the practice of peer review under the Health Care Quality Improvement Act of 1986 (42 U.S.C. §§11101 et seq.). This statute establishes peer review immunity from damage suits when the participants act in good faith in any peer review process that meets the act's standards for structure and fair process. Peer review is defined quite broadly, and protected participants include everyone involved in the process, from investigators to witnesses to medical peers.

STATUTORY PROTECTIONS SPECIFIC TO PARTICULAR REPORTING SYSTEMS

Some statutes have been crafted to protect specific reporting systems. Examples of these follow, along with some indications of their success in practice. All provide limited precedent for protecting data.

National Practitioner Data Bank (NPDB)

The federal Health Care Quality Improvement Act of 1986 (42 U.S.C. §§11101 et seq.) requires all malpractice insurers and self-insurers to report claims paid on behalf of named practitioners to the NPDB maintained by the Health Resources and Services Administration (HRSA). Decisions affecting clinical privileges of physicians and dentists must be reported by hospitals, state boards or professional associations; hospitals and other entities may voluntarily submit reports on other practitioners. Practitioners are also allowed limited space in the data bank to comment on the information reported (often asserting that the payment was made solely for tactical legal

---

*An unknown but key issue is the extent to which general harm to incentives to generate data would enter into a court's balancing.

reasons, not in recognition of medical failures). The reporting obligation is limited to specified formal determinations about consequential errors in medicine (claims settled, discipline meted out) and does not extend to simple observation of medical errors "in the field."

With regard to confidentiality, the act allows only designated authorized users to obtain information from the data bank, mainly hospitals and other health care organizations that credential practitioners. Regulations call for authorized users to use data only for credentialing or peer review and to keep data only within departments doing such authorized activities. The NPDB may not give information on any practitioner to any malpractice insurer, defense attorney, or member of the general public, although plaintiffs' attorneys may query the bank under very limited circumstances. Strong monetary penalties exist for unauthorized disclosures from the NPDB. Bills have often been filed in the Congress to "open up" the bank for public access, but these have always been opposed by federal authorities and have never been close to enactment. There is nonetheless substantial concern among practitioners that legislative change will eventually succeed.

Completeness of reporting is difficult to assess. Some physicians are said to avoid being reported to the data bank by settling lawsuits in the name of a corporate defendant and being dropped individually from the lawsuit. Insurers and corporate defendants, in turn, are said to report increased difficulty in settling claims because of the resistance of practitioners to being reported. HRSA sources interviewed said that they believe reporting is good, and said that occasional complaints referred to them almost always turn out to have been reported. HRSA interviewees said that there have been no known leaks from HRSA or from any contractor that has maintained the database. Complaints about leaks have been too general and non-specific to investigate.

The claims data in the data bank are effectively "protected" from discovery in a lawsuit involving the injury-producing error that was reported because the applicable lawsuit must already be over. Claim closure is what generates the duty to report, including information from the settlement. Plaintiffs might be interested in the data as similar-occurrence information, but no civil lawsuit subpoenas have been issued to the data bank; the protecting federal law preempts any attempts to obtain data for a state lawsuit. The NPDB does not face the problem of having to protect any investigators of reports, because it conducts no independent investigation, being prohibited by law from modifying information submitted in reports. Those who generate reports do face inquiries, however; when a physician is under review for privileges at a hospital, for example, the institution will routinely ask liability insurers and doctors about their reported history of malpractice and discipline, and no confidentiality applies.

Quality Improvement Organizations (QIOs)

Also known as peer review organizations (PROs), these entities monitor the utilization and quality of care for Medicare beneficiaries, including quality improvement projects, mandatory case review and oversight of program integrity (see Chapter 7). One responsibility involves the investigation and evaluation of instances of possibly substandard care provided to fee-for-service Medicare beneficiaries. Case review information with patient identifiers is not subject to subpoena in a civil action (42 CFR Section 476.140).

Veterans Health Administration System

The Veterans Health Administration (VHA) is planning to implement a voluntary, non-punitive reporting system on a pilot basis. This system is being designed after the aviation model (see Chapter 5) for eventual use throughout the VHA delivery system. A specific federal statute confers confidentiality for quality assurance within the VHA. The VHA's general counsel has not formally issued an opinion on whether the new reporting system will be protected by this statute, but VHA officials believe it will be. Because the system is not yet operational, there has been no opportunity for the statute's application to the reporting system to be challenged (the federal Tort Claims Act waives governmental immunity for the VHA, so it generally can be sued for medical malpractice).

Food and Drug Administration

Via its MedWatch system, the FDA receives reports from practitioners and manufacturers of serious adverse events and product problems related to medications and devices within its regulatory authority. Strict confidentiality rules apply to the identities of both reporters and patients; governing laws include the federal Privacy Act and the Freedom of Information Act. Agency regulations since 1995 have protected against disclosure of voluntary reports held by pharmaceutical, biological, and medical device manufacturers, by preempting state discovery laws.

New York Patient Occurrence Reporting and Tracking System

New York operates a leading example of a type of state regulatory system that collects reports of various types of adverse events. Access to individual reports is protected by statute. This statutory shield was challenged and was upheld by the courts, according to interviewees. Reports from hospitals are also protected by the statute protecting internal investigative reports and incident reports. If the department conducts an investigation of a specific event (prompted by a report or by a patient's complaint) official action is taken by the state (e.g., a statement of deficiencies), and the public and the patient have access to these findings. Accordingly, reporters can expect information reported to become public.

PRACTICAL PROTECTIONS AGAINST THE DISCOVERY OF DATA ON ERRORS

Two practical methods have been used to try to assure those who report errors that their reports will not be used in civil lawsuits against them or their colleagues. The first is simply to promise confidentiality by operational practice, but without full legal support in case of subpoena. Some organizations have tried to abide by a promise not to disclose the reporter's identity, and so far, have apparently been successful. However they appear to be vulnerable to subpoena.

The second practical protection is to obtain and maintain the data in a manner that prevents identification of the reporter or the specific event, even if a plaintiff obtains access to the report. This can be done with anonymous reporting (in which case the data recipient never receives any identified information to begin with) and by de-identification of reported data (in which case the identity of the reporter is removed after receipt of the report, often after a short lag to permit clarification or additional information to be obtained from the reporter). This section relates experience with these methods.

Confidentiality by Promise and Practice

A promise of confidentiality is sometimes the only option available to private organizations today. Two organizational examples are described below. Operational practice to maintain confidentiality can also be important within organizations that have dual roles—quality improvement and enforcement—so that the information on errors is sequestered behind an internal curtain of confidentiality and made available only to those who need access to it for purposes of analysis and prevention. Even such a "firewall" may not have credibility for reporters. The Aviation Safety Reporting System, for example, was not fully trusted by reporters until it was moved from within the Federal Aviation Administration (FAA) to a separate agency, the National Aeronautics and Space Administration (NASA).

JCAHO's sentinel event system is a notable example of confidentiality based on promise and practice. When first proposed in 1996, the policy caused controversy among hospitals fearful of disclosure to JCAHO. JCAHO has since changed its policy to permit hospitals to disclose details through on-site inspection by JCAHO investigators so that information stayed inside the institution and was not reported externally to JCAHO. One legal fear is that disclosure of internal quality data to outside reviewers not under a peer review statute will lead to discovery from JCAHO in lawsuits; indeed, many fear that disclosure to JCAHO would invalidate even the nondiscoverability protections each hospital enjoys for its own data under its state peer review statute.* A practical fear is that involving numerous outsiders will increase the potential for security breaches. JCAHO is seeking federal statutory protection as a definitive solution to the problem.

The Medical Error Reporting (MER) System also relies on a promise of confidentiality. It receives identified reports of medication errors, almost exclusively from practitioners. The reporter is given the option of not being identified to the sponsoring organizations (see Chapter 5), FDA, and the relevant pharmaceutical company, but the reporter's identity is maintained within the MER data system. Sometimes, anonymous reports are received. Lawyers have requested and been given copies of general reports on a particular problem, but not specific case reports. The data bank has never been subpoenaed, but the director considers this to be a significant risk that likely contributes to substantial under reporting.

Anonymous Reporting

The intent of anonymous reporting is to ensure that the reporter cannot be identified from the report. The information, therefore, can be used primarily as unidentified similar-occurrence data to prove particular aspects of

---

*The 50-state survey on peer review noted above was undertaken as part of the reaction against the initial JCAHO proposal for mandatory reporting of identified information.

a case, such as causation. The potential for this kind of generalized legal risk may not significantly deter reporting.

The use of anonymous reporting can reduce the effectiveness of the reporting system. On a practical level, a loss of information can occur because the data system is restricted to receive only the information transmitted initially by the reporter. The recipient cannot go back to the reporter to get clarification and additional information.

At a more fundamental level, some detailed information can be lost to the system because it might tend to identify the specific event or the reporter. This is especially true for injury-producing errors, because of the greater knowledge of the error possessed by a plaintiff compared with persons not involved in the event being reported. Plaintiffs know detailed information about their own cases that could enable each to identify with some certainty even an anonymous report or reporter about the specific injury being litigated. This information could include the dates of the event and the injury, nature and severity of the injury, type of facility, types of practitioners, and type and location of error. The names and types of specific equipment and drugs involved in the error, if any, also could help make the report identifiable to a plaintiff. As a result, information that is important to meet the needs of the reporting and analysis system might have to be omitted because it would serve to make the report identifiable to a plaintiff.

One example of an anonymous reporting system, is MedMARx. Hospitals submit reports on medication errors to MedMARx over the Internet, identified by a random number known only to the submitting hospital. This preserves anonymity, but allows the hospital to compare its experience to similar institutions. Because information is collected in a standardized format, the need to go back to the reporter for additional information is minimized. The usefulness of data for comparisons is enhanced by including "demographic" information on reporting hospitals (e.g., size, teaching status, location of error within hospital), but within categories sufficiently large to frustrate any attempt to identify reporters.

De-Identification

Two programs de-identify data as a practical protection against discovery. The Medical Event Reporting System for Transfusion Medicine (MERS-TM) is a private collaboration between blood centers and hospital transfusion services in Texas. Reports are generated within the protected quality assurance structures at each institution, but the Texas peer review statute may not apply to the data bank itself. Only near-miss data have been included to date, but the operators of the data bank are nonetheless extremely concerned about the possibility of receiving a subpoena. De-identification is the primary protection, but it causes them to lose information they would like to have about the reporting institution, such as the type of center, size, and location.

In the Aviation Safety Reporting System (ASRS), the reporter's name and contact information are retained temporarily in case additional information is needed. De-identification usually occurs within 72 hours of the initial receipt of the report. There has been no breach of identity of the reporter in more than 20 years of operation.

SUMMARY

Litigators have strong incentives and powerful legal tools to obtain information about errors to assist them in lawsuits for medical injuries. Many reporting systems contain information that would be useful to plaintiffs. The more that the content of a particular reporting system resembles the claims files of a medical liability insurer, the more attractive a target reporting system is for the plaintiffs. For example, a reporting system that focuses only on identified injury-causing errors from a small number of institutions is more attractive to plaintiffs than one that collects large numbers of nonidentified near misses from many different types of reporters in different states.

Fear of legal discoverability or involvement in the legal process is believed to contribute to underreporting of errors. Collaborative quality improvement efforts may be inhibited by the loss of statutory peer review protection that may occur when data are shared across institutions. Some form of protection appears necessary for each of the three components of an error reporting system: (1) the original reporters; (2) the various recipients of the information (including processors, investigators, de-identifiers, and analyzers); and (3) the reported information itself. Information voluntarily shared should be done with appropriate safeguards for patient confidentiality.

Legal protections are the only possible way to protect identified reporters, report recipients, and reports from discovery but legal protections are not without problems. Specific statutory protection for a particular reporting system may be the most desirable form of protection, but this may not be a realistic option for many systems. Some states' peer review statutes could be used by some types of reporting systems—for example in California and

Oklahoma—but the assurance of protection is not ironclad. Other states' statutes would need revision to accommodate external data banks and collaborative efforts. This would require careful drafting that could survive state-by-state political processes, with careful attention to the scope of the protection, definitions of authorized users and uses, potential loopholes, and the like.

A more promising alternative, proposed recently by the Medicare Payment Advisory Commission (1999), is for Congress to enact protective federal legislation.[29] Such legislation could be enacted immediately and would not rely on actions to be taken by 50 different states.

Practical methods can be very useful in protecting nonidentified *reporters*, *recipients*, and *reported data*, but they also have some weaknesses, so reporters may not fully trust them. The level of protection of practical methods differs somewhat for the three components of reporting systems. *Reporters* could be protected from subpoena if all potentially identifying information is absent from the report, but anonymous reporting and de-identification may not be effective if the likely reporter can be identified readily by the plaintiff independent of the reports. This may occur, for example, when only one person is the logical or mandated reporter for an organization or department within the organization.

Similarly, *recipients* of reports (processors, investigators, etc.) might become identifiable to a plaintiff. A recipient who handles large numbers of reports may not remember details about any specific report. However, if an investigator spent some time on-site looking into a particular event, as might a JCAHO investigator examining a hospital's root cause analysis of a particular sentinel event, practical methods of protection would likely fail.

Any *reported data* of an injury-causing error can be protected from use in a lawsuit involving that specific reported injury by practical methods (anonymous reporting or de-identification). In nonidentified form, the report might still be useful to plaintiffs in other cases as a similar occurrence, but whether this type of use would deter reporting is an empirical question that might vary with the reporting system and might change over time. In addition, anonymous reporting and de-identified reporting both cause reports to lose some information. The information loss would likely be greatest for reports of injury-producing errors, which an informed plaintiff might seek.

Legal protections may help patch up the weaknesses of practical methods of protection. Depending on the nature of the reporting system (geographic catchment, type of reporters, number and type of events reported), legal protection may be a necessary supplement to practical protections for possibly identifiable reporters, recipients, and reports. Supplementary legal protection also could ameliorate the loss of data that might otherwise occur to preserve nonidentifiability. If legal use of similar-occurrence data does in fact deter reporting, then legal protection may be desirable to prevent even this type of use. The strongest legal protections would cover the entire chain of custody of the information, from its initial generation to its ultimate use. This strong form of protection is used, for example, in the Health Care Quality Improvement Act's protection for the peer review process.

The committee concludes that some combination of legal and practical protections would be best. Each alone is imperfect, but they are mutually reinforcing and together can provide the strongest assurance of confidentiality.

REFERENCES

1. Steves, Myron F. A Proposal to Improve the Cost to Benefit Relationships in the Medical Professional Liability Insurance System. *Duke Law Journal.* 16:1305–1333, 1975.

2. Abraham, Kenneth S. and Weiler, Paul C. Enterprise Medical Liability and the Evolution of the American Health Care System. *Harv L Rev.* 108:381, 1994.

3. Sage, William M.; Hastings, K. E.; Berenson, Robert A. Enterprise Liability for Medical Malpractice and Health Care Quality Improvement. *Am J Law Med.* 20:1–28, 1994.

4. Bovbjerg, Randall R. and Sloan, Frank A. A No Fault for Medical Injury: Theory and Evidence. *University of Cincinnati Law Review.* 67:53–123, 1998.

5. Many lessons from Workers' Compensation and one limited medical no-fault approach are set out in Bovbjerg and Sloan, 1998.

6. Federal Rule of Evidence 401: "Relevant evidence means evidence having any tendency to make the existence of any fact that is of consequence to the determination of the action more probable or less probable than it would be without the evidence."

7. Weinstein's Federal Evidence 2nd ed., 1998, Vol. 2, Section 401.03.

8. Weinstein's Federal Evidence, 2nd ed., 1998, Vol. 2, Section 401.07.

9. Federal Rule of Evidence 402.

10. Ziegler v. Superior Court of County of Pima (1982, app) 134 Ariz. 390, 656 P2d 1251. In this case, the names of the patients were removed to protect their privacy.

11. Amente v. Newman 653 So 2d 1030, 20 FLW S172 (1995, Fla).

12. Moore, James W.; Vestal, Allan D.; and Kurland, Phillip B. Moore's Manual: Federal Practice and Procedure. 2(15):03[2][a], 1998.

13. "The information sought need not be admissible at the trial if the information sought appears reasonably calculated to lead to the discovery of admissible evidence." Federal Rule of Civil Procedure 26(b).

14. Federal Rule of Civil Procedure 45.

15. Rhode Island Rule of Evidence 407.

16. Fox v. Kramer (Calif. 6th App. Dist. 1999) 1999 Daily Journal D.A.R. 1772.

17. Leonard, David R., New Wigmore's Treatise on Evidence: Selected Rules of Limited Admissibility, Ch. 2, 1999 Suppl., Section 2:46–1.

18. Federal Rule of Evidence 407.

19. Leonard, David R., New Wigmore's Treatise on Evidence: Selected Rules of Limited Admissibility, Ch. 2, Supp., Section 2:46–51, 1999.

20. State ex rel. United Hospital Center, Inc. v. Bedell (W. Va. 1997) 484 SE2d 199; Columbia/HCA Healthcare Corporation v. Eighth Judicial District Court, (Nev. 1997) 936 P2d 844.

21. Columbia/HCA Healthcare Corporation v. Eighth Judicial District Court, (Nev. 1997) 936 P2d 844.

22. Brennan, Elise D. Peer Review Confidentiality. American Health Lawyers Association Annual Meeting, 1998.

23. Mills, D. H. Medical Peer Review: The Need to Organize a Protective Approach. *Health Matrix.* 1(1):67–76, 1991.

24. Mills, 1991.

25. California Business and Professions Code Section 805.

26. City of Edmond v. Parr, 1978 OK 70, 578 P.2d 56 (Okla. 1978).

27. Arnett v. Dal Cielo, 42 Cal. Rptr. 2d 712 (1995); Arizona Occupations Code Section 32-1451.01(E).

28. West Covina Hospital v. Superior Court, 41 Cal. 3d 846, 718 P. 2d. 119 (1986).

29. See Medicare Payment Advisory Commission (1999), recommendation 3C, at p. 36.

BIBLIOGRAPHY

ASRS (Aviation Safety Reporting System). 1999. Program Overview. http://olias.arc.nasa.gov/asrs/Overview.html accessed 28 July 1999.

Berwick, Donald. M. Continuous Improvement as an Ideal in Health Care. *N Engl J Med.* 320:53–56, 1989.

Bodenheimer, Thomas. The American Health Care System—The Movement for Improved Quality in Health Care. *N Engl J Med.* 340(6):488–492, 1999.

Brown, Lowell C. and Meinhardt, Robyn. Peer Review Confidentiality: Those Old Protections Just Ain't What They Used to Be. *Whittier Law Review.* 18:99–104, 1996.

Bovbjerg, Randall R. and Sloan, Frank A. No Fault for Medical Injury: Theory and Evidence. *University of Cincinnati Law Review.* 67:53–123, 1998.

Friend, Gail N., et al. The New Rules of Show and Tell: Identifying and Protecting the Peer Review and Medical Committee Privileges. *Baylor Law Review.* 49:607–656, 1997.

Joint Commission on the Accreditation of Healthcare Organizations. Sentinel Event Policy and Procedures, 1998. http://wwwa.jcaho.org/ns-search/sentinel/se_poly.htm?NS-search-set=/36c06/aaaa17864c065ea&NS-doc-offset=0& accessed February 9, 1999.

Kutrow, Bradley. Accident Reports Take on New Status with North Carolina Court Ruling. *The Business Journal of Charlotte,* June 1, 1998. http://www.amcity.com/charlotte/stories/060198/smallb4.html accessed January 19, 1999.

Leape, Lucian. Error in Medicine. *JAMA*. 272:1851–1857, 1994.

Leape, Lucian L.; Woods, David D.; Hatlie, Martin J., et al. Promoting patient safety by preventing medical error. *JAMA*. 280:1444–1447, 1998.

Liang, Bryan A. Error in Medicine: Legal Impediments to U.S. Reform. *J Health Polit Policy Law*. 24:27–58, 1999.

Medicare Payment Advisory Commission. Report to the Congress: Selected Medicare Issues. Washington, DC: MedPAC, June, 1999.

National Patient Safety Foundation. Diverse Groups Come Together to Improve Health care Safety Through the National Patient Safety Foundation. Press Release August 29, 1997 <http://www.ama-assn.org/med-sci/npsf/pr897.htm>.

Pape, Julie Barker. Physician Data Banks: The Public's Right to Know Versus the Physician's Right to Privacy. *Fordham Law Review*. 66:975–1028, 1997.

Smarr, Lawrence E. A Comparative Assessment of the PIAA Data Sharing Project and the National Practitioner Data Bank: Policy, Purpose, and Application. *Law and Cont Prob*. 60(1):59–79, 1997.

Weiler, Paul C.; Newhouse, Joseph P.; and Hiatt, Howard H. Proposal for Medical Liability Reform. *JAMA*. 267:2355–2358, 1992.

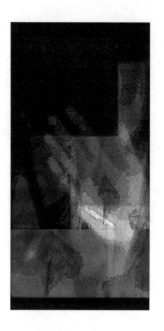

7
Setting Performance Standards and Expectations for Patient Safety

The development and availability of standards for patient safety can serve several purposes. They can either establish minimum levels of performance or can establish consistency or uniformity across multiple individuals and organizations. Another purpose for standards is that they set expectations. The process of developing standards can set expectations for the organizations and health professionals affected by the standards. The publication and dissemination of standards additionally helps to set expectations for consumers and purchasers.

Standards can be developed and used in public regulatory processes, such as licensure for health professionals and licensure for health care organizations, such as hospitals or health plans. Standards can also be developed through private voluntary processes, such as professional certification or organizational accreditation.

Although there are many kinds of standards in health care, especially those promulgated by licensing agencies and accrediting organizations, few standards focus explicitly on issues of patient safety. Furthermore, the current lack of safety standards does not allow consumers and purchasers to reinforce the need for safe systems from the providers and organizations with whom they have contact. All existing regulatory and voluntary standard-setting organizations can increase their attention to patient safety and should consistently reinforce its importance.

Expectations for the performance of health professionals and organizations are also shaped by professional groups, purchasers and consumers, and society in general. Professional groups and leaders play a particularly important role in establishing norms and facilitating improvements in performance through educational, convening and advocacy activities. Large public and private group purchasers and purchasing coalitions also have the opportunity to shape expectations through marketplace decisions.

This chapter describes how performance standards and expectations can foster improvements in patient safety. Although this report has described the importance of a systems approach for reducing errors in health care, licensing and accreditation of individual practitioners and organizations can also play a role in reinforcing the importance of patient safety. The primary focus is on how existing models of oversight can be strengthened to include a focus on patient safety. In this report, the committee did not undertake an evaluation of the effectiveness of public and private oversight systems to affect quality of care. The committee recognizes, however, that as the organizational arrangements through which health care is delivered change, an evaluation may be appropriate since the existing models of oversight may no longer be adequate.

RECOMMENDATIONS

In the health care industry, standards and expectations about performance are applicable to health care organizations, health professionals, and drugs and devices. The committee believes there are numerous opportunities to strengthen the focus of the existing processes on patient safety issues.

RECOMMENDATION 7.1 Performance standards and expectations for heath care organizations should focus greater attention on patient safety.

- **Regulators and accreditors should require health care organizations to implement meaningful patient safety programs with defined executive responsibility.**
- **Public and private purchasers should provide incentives to health care organizations to demonstrate continuous improvement in patient safety.**

Changes within health care organizations will have the most direct impact on making care delivery processes safer for patients. Regulators and accreditors have a role in encouraging and supporting actions within health care organizations by holding them accountable for ensuring a safe environment for patients.

Health care organizations ought to be developing patient safety programs within their own organizations (see Chapter 8). After a reasonable period of time for health care organizations to set up such programs, regulators and accreditors should require patient safety programs as a minimum standard. The marketplace, through purchaser and consumer demands, also exerts influence on health care organizations. Public and private purchasers have three tools that can be employed today to demand better attention to safety by health care organizations. First, purchasers can consider safety issues in their contracting decisions. Second, purchasers can reinforce the importance of patient safety by providing relevant information to their employees or beneficiaries. There is increasing attention in providing information to aid in the selection of health coverage. Information about safety can be part of that process. Finally, purchasers can communicate concerns about patient safety to accrediting bodies to support stronger oversight for patient safety.

RECOMMENDATION 7.2 Performance standards and expectations for health professionals should focus greater attention on patient safety.

- **Health professional licensing bodies should**

(1)   implement periodic reexaminations and relicensing of doctors, nurses, and other key providers, based on both competence and knowledge of safety practices; and
(2)   work with certifying and credentialing organizations to develop more effective methods to identify unsafe providers and take action.

- **Professional societies should make a visible commitment to patient safety by establishing a permanent committee dedicated to safety improvement. This committee should**

(1)   develop a curriculum on patient safety and encourage its adoption into training and certification requirements;
(2)   disseminate information on patient safety to members at special sessions at annual conferences, journal articles and editorials, newsletters, publications and websites on a regular basis;

(3) recognize patient safety considerations in practice guidelines and in standards related to the introduction and diffusion of new technologies, therapies, and drugs;
(4) work with the Center for Patient Safety to develop community-based, collaborative initiatives for error reporting and analysis and implementation of patient safety improvements; and
(5) collaborate with other professional societies and disciplines in a national summit on the professional's role in patient safety.

For most health professionals, current methods of licensing and credentialing assess knowledge, but do not assess performance skills after initial licensure. Although the state grants initial licensure, responsibility for documenting continued competence is dispersed. Competence may be considered when a licensing board reacts to a complaint. It may be evaluated when an individual applies to a health care organization for privileges or network contracting or employment. Professional certification is the current process for evaluating clinical knowledge after licensure and some programs are now starting to consider assessment of clinical skills in addition to clinical knowledge. Given the rapid pace of change in health care and the constant development of new technologies and information, existing licensing and accreditation processes should be strengthened to ensure that all health care professionals are assessed periodically on both skills and knowledge for practice.

More effective methods for identifying unsafe providers and better coordination between the organizations involved are also needed. The time between discovery of a problem, investigation, and action can currently last several years, depending on the issue and procedures for appeal or other processes. Efforts should be made to make this time as short as possible, while ensuring that practitioners have available the due process procedures to which they are entitled. States should also be more active in notifying other states when a practitioner's license is rescinded. Although unsafe practitioners are believed to be few in number and efforts to identify such individuals are not likely to improve overall quality or safety problems throughout the industry, such efforts are important to a comprehensive safety program.

Finally, professional societies and groups should become active leaders in encouraging and demanding improvements in patient safety. Setting standards, convening and communicating with members about safety, incorporating attention to patient safety into training programs, and collaborating across disciplines are all mechanisms that will contribute to creating a culture of safety. As patient advocates, health care professionals owe their patients nothing less.

RECOMMENDATION 7.3 The Food and Drug Administration (FDA) should increase attention to the safe use of drugs in both pre- and postmarketing processes through the following actions:

- **develop and enforce standards for the design of drug packaging and labeling that will maximize safety in use;**
- **require pharmaceutical companies to test (using FDA-approved methods) proposed drug names to identify and remedy potential sound-alike and look-alike confusion with existing drug names; and**
- **work with physicians, pharmacists, consumers and others to establish appropriate responses to problems identified through postmarketing surveillance, especially for concerns that are perceived to require immediate response to protect the safety of patients.**

FDA's role is to regulate manufacturers for the safety of their drugs and devices; however, even approved drugs can present safety problems when used in practice. Drugs may be prone to error in use due to sound-alike or look-alike names, unclear labeling, or poorly designed packaging. FDA standards for packaging and labeling of drugs should consider the safety of the products in actual use. Manufacturers should also be required to use proven methods for detecting drug names that sound or look similar. If necessary, Congress should take appropriate action to provide additional enabling authority or clarification of existing authority for FDA to implement this action. Since not all safety problems can be predicted or avoided before a drug is marketed, FDA should also conduct intensive and extensive monitoring to identify problems early and respond quickly when serious threats are discovered in the actual use of approved drugs.

CURRENT APPROACHES FOR SETTING STANDARDS IN HEALTH CARE

Generically, standards can be used to define a process or outcome of care. The Institute of Medicine defines a quality standard as a minimum level of acceptable performance or results or excellent levels of performance or results or the range of acceptable performance or results.[1] Other definitions for standards have been enacted through legislation, such as the Occupational Safety and Health Act of 1970, which defines a safety and health standard as one that requires conditions, or the adoption or use of one or more practices, means, methods, operations or processes, reasonably necessary or appropriate to provide safe or healthful employment and places of employment.[2] A variety of standards have also been defined through private organizations, such as the American Society for Testing and Materials (see Appendix B). The committee does not recommend one definition or type of standard over another, but recognizes that standards can be quite varied and that as standards specific to safety are developed, they could take multiple forms and focus.

In health care, standards are set through both public, regulatory initiatives and private, voluntary initiatives. Standards can apply to health care organizations, health professionals, and drugs and medical devices. For health care organizations (e.g., health plans, hospitals, ambulatory care facilities), standards are set through licensure and accreditation and, to some extent, requirements imposed by large purchasers, such as Medicare and Fortune 500 companies. For health care professionals, standards are set through state licensure, board certification, and accrediting and credentialing programs. For drugs and devices, the FDA plays a critical role in standard setting.

In general, current standards in health care do not provide adequate focus on patient safety. Organizational licensure and accreditation focus on the review of core processes such as credentialing, quality improvement, and risk management, but lack a specific focus on patient safety issues. Professional licensure concentrates on qualifications at initial licensure, with no requirements to demonstrate safe and competent clinical skills during one's career. Standards for drugs and medical devices concentrate on safe design and production, with less attention to their safe use. Current standards in health care leave serious gaps in ensuring patient safety.

PERFORMANCE STANDARDS AND EXPECTATIONS FOR HEALTH CARE ORGANIZATIONS

Standards and expectations for health care organizations may be established through oversight processes, primarily licensing and accreditation requirements. Additionally, large public and private purchasers may also impose demands on health care organizations. Each is discussed in this section.

Licensing and Accreditation

There is a great deal of variation in state licensure requirements for health care organizations. Responsibility for licensure rests at the state level, with each state setting its own standards, measurement, and enforcement. Although standards and measurement can be made more similar, enforcement is always likely to vary to some extent depending on the level of resources devoted by a state to this activity.

In many states, licensure and accreditation are intertwined. For hospital licensure, 44 states accept the Joint Commission on Accreditation of Healthcare Organization's evaluation, in whole or in part, as a condition for licensure (Margaret VanAmringe, JCAHO, personal communication, February 23, 1999). Some states may additionally require compliance with other standards related to building safety or medical care issues that are tracked in that particular state. The remaining states do not link hospital licensure and accreditation. Although the overwhelming tendency to use JCAHO increases the consistency of standards nationally, differences in application also contribute to the variation in ensuring patient safety. For licensure of health maintenance organizations (HMOs), some states rely on private accrediting bodies, primarily the National Committee for Quality Assurance (NCQA), to conduct reviews of health plans. It should also be noted that other health facilities, such as some ambulatory care centers or physicians' offices, may not be licensed at all and are generally not subject to traditional methods of oversight. One of the few mechanisms in place today that more broadly examines care in the ambulatory setting is managed care organizations.

Three private-sector agencies play a role in organizational accreditation: JCAHO, NCQA, and the American Accreditation Healthcare Commission/ URAC. Each effort, to some degree, encompasses aspects of standard setting and performance measurement.

JCAHO accredits more than 18,000 health care organizations, including hospitals, health plans, home care agencies, and others.[3] Its longest-standing accreditation program applies to hospitals. JCAHO accredits hospitals for three-year periods based on compliance with its standards in the areas of patient rights and patient care: organizational performance; leadership; information management; and nursing and medical staff structures. Approximately 85 percent of hospitals are accredited by JCAHO. Both Joint Commission-accredited hospitals and those accredited by the American Osteopathic Association are deemed to meet Medicare conditions of participation. JCAHO is incorporating performance information into the accreditation process through its Oryx system, in which hospitals will collect clinical data on six measures and submit performance data on these measures. This system was introduced in 1997 and is required by the Joint Commission for a hospital to be accredited. Eventually hospitals will have to demonstrate specific Oryx performance to maintain their accreditation status.

NCQA accredits health plans for periods of one, two, or three years. The accreditation process covers areas related to quality improvement, credentialing, members' rights and responsibilities, preventive health services, utilization management, and medical records. Approximately 14 states incorporate accreditation into their licensure requirement for health plans; another six states require that health plans have external reviews, most of which are done by NCQA (Steve Lamb, NCQA, personal communication, March 2, 1999). A number of states also require that health plans serving public employees and/or Medicaid enrollees be accredited. NCQA's performance dataset, the Health Plan Employer Data and Information Set (HEDIS), looks at indicators of effectiveness of care, access or availability, satisfaction, health plan stability, use of services, and costs. Beginning in July 1999, accreditation criteria began to incorporate HEDIS measures, initially being used only if they increase a health plan's overall score.[4] Accreditation status will also change with the top 20 percent of health plans earning the status of "excellent."

URAC was established in 1990 and offers nine different accreditation programs for managed care organizations, such as health plan accreditation, health network accreditation, health utilization management accreditation, and network practitioner credentialing.[5] Individual managed care organizations can seek accreditation under different sets of programs depending on the range of services they offer. URAC accreditation focuses on preferred provider organization (PPO) and point-of-service (POS) plans. Approximately 22 states have incorporated Commission/URAC accreditation into their regulatory structures.

Purchaser Requirements and Demands

Both private and public purchasers have the ability to encourage health care organizations and providers to pursue continuous improvements in patient safety. Large group purchasers, such as Fortune 500 companies or the Health Care Financing Administration, and purchasing coalitions that provide insurance to large numbers of people are well positioned to exert considerable leverage in the marketplace.

Private Group Purchasers

There are numerous examples of large private employers that incorporate quality issues into their decision-making process when selecting health plans and providers to offer to employees.[6] Xerox Corporation ranks health plans according to various quality indicators, including accreditation status, satisfaction ratings, and quality indicators. ARCO evaluates health plans based on 50 different quality and access criteria, and ties the employer contribution to the premium level of the highest-ranking plan. In a survey of 33 large purchasers in four states, 45 percent reported using HEDIS data (i.e., NCQA's Healthplan Employer Data and Information Set quality indicators), 55 percent reported using accreditation data, and 53 percent reported using consumer satisfaction survey data to choose a health plan.[7]

Although some large employers have incorporated quality considerations into their purchasing decisions, this is not the norm. A 1997 survey of 325 U.S. companies found that most employers consider provider network characteristics, but only a fraction consider quantifiable measures of access, quality or outcomes.[8] Another survey found that nearly two-thirds of midsize and large employers are unfamiliar with NCQA accreditation, the most widely used accreditation program for health plans.[9]

Clearly, there is much opportunity for large employers to place greater emphasis on quality, and specifically patient safety, issues when making decisions to contract with a specific health plan and in the design of payment and financial incentive systems to reward demonstrated quality and safety improvements.

Health Care Financing Administration

As a major national purchaser of health care services, HCFA sets standards through payment policies and conditions of participation for the organizations with which it contracts. HCFA provides health insurance for 74 million people through Medicare, and in partnership with the states, Medicaid, and Child Health Insurance programs.[10] It also performs a number of quality-focused activities, including regulation of laboratory testing, surveys and certification, development of coverage policies, and quality improvement initiatives.

The peer review organizations (PROs) monitor the utilization and quality of care of Medicare beneficiaries through a state-based network.[11] They have three functions. First, they conduct cooperative quality improvement projects in partnership with other quality-focused organizations. Among the current projects are programs on diabetes, end-stage renal disease, influenza campaign, and quality improvement systems for managed care. Second, PROs conduct mandatory case review in response to beneficiary complaints, as well as educational and outreach activities. Third, they oversee program integrity by ensuring that Medicare pays only for medically necessary services. Patient safety has not been identified as a priority to date, however, HCFA is giving serious consideration to making patient safety a higher priority.[12]

Medicare and Medicaid survey and certification activities are aimed at ensuring that providers and suppliers for these programs meet health, safety, and program standards.[13] They deal with issues related to the effective and efficient delivery of care to beneficiaries, ensuring their safety while in health care facilities and improving their quality of care. HCFA relies on state health agencies as the principal agents to perform certification activities through their licensure activities. As already noted, state health departments, in turn, often rely on JCAHO as part of licensing a hospital.

STANDARDS FOR HEALTH PROFESSIONALS

Performance standards and expectations for health professionals may be defined through regulatory and other oversight processes, such as licensing, accreditation, and certification. Standards and expectations may also be shaped by professional societies and other groups that voluntarily promulgate guidelines or protocols and sponsor educational and convening activities.

Licensing, Certification, and Accreditation

Compared to facility licensure (as discussed in the previous section) there is even greater variation found in professional licensure. There are several reasons for this. First, professional licensure is structured through individual licensing boards for each regulated profession in the state.[14] The result is variation both within states and across states. Within states, there is little coordination of management or dissemination of information among different boards.[15] Across states, there is variation in what is considered a complaint and in the rate at which disciplinary action is taken. Variation in what is considered a "complaint" influences what is investigated and what can be shared and when. A call to the licensing board may be considered a complaint, or a complaint may be recognized only when there is a formal charge. It is not clear, therefore, when information can be shared: when something is filed (which may or may not lead to a charge), while it is being investigated, after there is a charge, or only if disciplinary action is taken. Inconsistencies permit unsafe practitioners to move to different jurisdictions before a complaint can be investigated and handled.[16]

Although not a comprehensive measure of effectiveness, there is wide variation in the rate at which state licensing boards take serious disciplinary actions against physicians, ranging from 0.85 per 1,000 physicians in Louisiana to 15.40 per 1,000 physicians in Alaska, based on data from the Federation of State Medical Boards.[17] Across the country, the rate was 3.76 actions per 1,000 physicians in 1998. States that appeared to be doing a better job (more disciplinary actions) tended to have better funding, and more staff, conducted proactive investigations (as opposed to waiting for complaints), used other available data (e.g., Medicare or Medicaid data), had good leadership, were independent from state medical societies and other parts of state government, and had a reasonable statutory framework for conducting their work. Board action can also be quite slow. For example, the Virginia Board of Medicine takes an average of more than two and a half years to resolve a case.[18]

The National Council of State Boards of Nursing has endorsed a mutual recognition model for interstate nursing practice to encourage reciprocal arrangements between states for licensing and disciplinary action (Carolyn Hutcherson, National Council of State Boards of Nursing, personal communication, June 1, 1999).[19] The goal would be to make licensure more like the rules used for a driver's license. That is, licensure is recognized across state lines, but the nurse would still be subject to the rules of a state while in that state (e.g., even if a driver's residence is in Maryland, the driver can still get a speeding ticket in Texas).

Another issue related to professional licensure is that there is no continuing assessment or required demonstration of performance after initial licensure is granted, except for physician assistants and emergency medical technicians.[20] In general, the state is involved in initial licensure or follow-up of complaints; processes for documenting continued competence are voluntary.

For example, physicians may voluntarily seek board certification through one of 24 specialty medical boards that have been approved by the American Board of Medical Specialties (ABMS).[21] The specialty boards set professional and educational standards for the evaluation and certification of physician specialists. Initial certification is granted by passing written and oral examinations. Recertification occurs at seven- to ten-year intervals, although not all boards require recertification. Recertification is granted based on self-assessment, examinations, and credentialing (e.g., unrestricted license, good standing in practice, hospital privileges (Linda Blank, American Board of Internal Medicine, personal communication, May 18, 1999). A minimum number of continuing education credits may also be required. At the present time, there is no assessment of practice skills, although some specialty boards have committed a broader and more timely assessment of competence.[22]

Another voluntary approach is the American Medical Accreditation Program (AMAP), which is being developed by the American Medical Association. AMAP is a voluntary process, begun in 1998, for the accreditation of individual physicians that is designed to measure and evaluate individual physicians against national standards and peer performance.[23] The program will evaluate physicians in five areas: (1) credentials; (2) personal qualifications (including ethical behavior and participation in continuing medical education, peer reviews, and self-assessment of performance); (3) environment of care (including a site review of office operations and medical records); (4) clinical processes (including standardized measures of key patient care processes and comparative feedback to the physician); and (5) patient outcomes (including standardized measures of patient outcomes, perceptions of care, and health status). Although this is a national program, it is being implemented on a state-by-state basis.

A comparable process is found in nursing, which recognizes specialty practice through board certification. One such specialty certifying body is the American Nurses Credentialing Center (ANCC), a subsidiary of the American Nurses Association. Specialty certifying boards set professional and educational standards for the defined specialty and determine a mechanism for establishing continued competency through the recertification process, which occurs every three to five years, depending on the specialty. Although safety is not an explicit focus of certification exams, areas covered may relate to safety, for example, medication errors. Nurses may pursue certification voluntarily, although some states require it for licensure at advanced levels such as nurse practitioner (Ann Carey, R.N., American Nurses Credentialing Center, personal communication, July 20, 1999). Certifying organizations are exploring alternative ways to validate continued competency in addition to continuing education.

Health care organizations are also involved in assessing the continued performance of professionals when hiring nurses or credentialing physicians for hospital privileges, network membership, or employment. Again, there is little consistency in the standards used and little opportunity for communication across organizations. For example, an unsafe provider may be dismissed from one hospital, with no notification to the licensing board and limited ability for the next hospital to find out the reasons for the dismissal.

The Pew Health Professions Commission conducted an extensive investigation of licensure and continued competency issues. Its report identifies four places in which assessment of competency can occur: upon entry into practice, for continuing authorization to practice, reentry to practice, and after disciplinary action.[24] The report recommended increased state regulation to require health care practitioners to "demonstrate their competence in the knowledge, judgment, technical skills and interpersonal skills relevant to their jobs throughout their career." They note that considerations of competence should include not only the basic and specialized knowledge and skills, but also other skills such as "capacity to admit errors." In their view, the current system that relies on continuing education and disciplinary action after a problem has occurred is insufficient. The trend toward computer-based testing should facilitate greater attention to skill assessment in the future. Physician licensure tests and physician recertification are moving toward interactive, computer-based testing, and nursing is also testing a computerized system for initial licensure.[25]

The Role of Health Professional Societies and Groups

Professional societies, groups, and associations can play an important role in improving patient safety by contributing to the creation of a culture that encourages the identification and prevention of errors. Few professional societies or groups have demonstrated a visible commitment to reducing errors in health care and improving patient safety. Although it is believed that the commitment exists among their members, there has been little collective action. The exception most often cited is the work that has been done by anesthesiologists to improve safety and outcomes for patients.

Anesthesiology has successfully reduced anesthesia mortality rates from two deaths per 10,000 anesthetics administered to one death per 200,000–300,000 anesthetics administered (see Chapter 2). This success was accomplished through a combination of:

- technological changes (new monitoring equipment, standardization of existing equipment);

- information-based strategies, including the development and adoption of guidelines and standards;
- application of human factors to improve performance, such as the use of simulators for training;
- formation of the Anesthesia Patient Safety Foundation to bring together stakeholders from different disciplines (physicians, nurses, manufacturers) to create a focus for action; and
- having a leader who could serve as a champion for the cause.[26]

To explore the ways that professional societies could improve patient safety, the Institute of Medicine (IOM) convened a one-day workshop on September 9, 1999 with 14 health professionals representing medicine, nursing, and pharmacy (workshop participants are included in the acknowledgments). These leaders are interested and involved in issues related to patient safety and are active in professional societies, although they did not participate in the workshop as representatives of these societies. Four broad roles were identified that could be employed, individually or in combination, to create a culture of safety. These roles are: (1) defining standards of practice; (2) convening and collaborating among society members and with other groups; (3) encouraging research, training and education opportunities; and (4) advocating for change.

One way that professional societies contribute to standards of practice is through the promulgation and promotion of practice guidelines. A number of professional groups have produced practice guidelines and defined best practices in select areas. Guidelines produced by the American College of Cardiology (ACC) and the American Heart Association Task Force of Practice Guidelines are consistently cited models. They have produced sixteen guidelines ranging from coronary artery bypass graft (CABG) to management of chronic angina.[27]

Pharmacy has also devoted significant attention to patient safety. The American Society of Health-System Pharmacists (ASHP) has published extensively on safe medication practices. Reduction of medication errors has been an identified priority for a decade and is reflected through publications in professional and scientific journals, educational programming, and advocacy. Included among the standards and guidelines is a widely disseminated list of the top priority actions for preventing adverse drug events in hospitals.

Practice guidelines can also be written through a more interdisciplinary approach, such as the perinatal guidelines published jointly by the American

College of Obstetricians and Gynecologists (ACOG) and the American Academy of Pediatrics. There is now a fourth edition of these guidelines. As recognition has grown that errors are caused by failures in systems, interdisciplinary collaboration may become increasingly necessary for redesigning complex systems of care. Participants at the workshop suggested that professional societies develop guidelines devoted specifically to patient safety and the incorporation of patient safety considerations into other guidelines.

One of the most visible activities of professional groups is their convening function. Through annual conferences and specialty meetings, professional groups can develop and communicate standards, values, and policy statements to membership and key opinion leaders. Meeting conclusions may also be disseminated through their own and other journal publications. There are few examples of specialty meetings or conferences where patient safety has been explicitly included on the agenda. Additionally, there are few interdisciplinary conferences devoted to issues of patient safety. Participants at the workshop proposed a national conference that would bring together all health professions and professionals from other disciplines (e.g., industrial engineering, human factors analysis) and other industries (e.g., airline pilots).

Clinical training and education is a key mechanism for cultural change. Colleges of medicine, nursing, pharmacy, health care administration, and their related associations should build more instruction into their curriculum on patient safety and its relationship to quality improvement. One of the challenges in accomplishing this is the pressure on clinical education programs to incorporate a broadening array of topics. Many believe that initial exposure to patient safety should occur early in undergraduate and graduate training programs, as well as through continuing education. Clinical training programs also need to ensure that teaching opportunities are safe for patients. One workshop participant told of a monitoring device used to alert staff to possible problems with the patient that was turned off because it was seen as interfering with the teaching experience.

The need for more opportunities for interdisciplinary training was also identified. Most care delivered today is done by teams of people, yet training often remains focused on individual responsibilities leaving practitioners inadequately prepared to enter complex settings. Improving patient safety also requires some understanding of systems theory in order to effectively analyze the many contributing factors that influence errors. Again, the "silos" created through training and organization of care impede safety improvements. Instruction in safety improvement requires knowledge about working in teams, using information and information technology, quality measurement, and communicating with patients about errors. A background in other disciplines is also relevant, such as cognitive psychology, systems theory, and statistics.[28] Principles of crew resource management used to train personnel who work together in airline cockpits might also be applicable to health care. Training should also emphasize better communications across disciplines. This is important when the members of a care team are in one physical location, such as a hospital or office setting, but becomes even more important when the care team may not be in one place, such as a team providing home care.

Few professional groups have sufficient resources to devote to research support, although many have established research and education foundations. The need for greater collaboration in developing regional databases was noted. A key advantage of establishing these at the regional level is the ability to obtain a sufficient number of cases for meaningful analysis. The number of cases of any particular event in a single hospital or clinical setting is usually too small to be able to generalize across cases and identify a way to make system improvements. Regional data systems can increase numbers to improve analytic power and can facilitate collaboration to understand the extent and nature of errors in health care. Professional societies and groups could participate in efforts to coordinate a research agenda and the development of databases to provide information on the extent and nature of errors in health care.

Professional groups can also serve as advocates for change. Professional groups have been able to call attention to a health risk and create awareness. For example, pediatricians have been active in promoting increased immunization rates, the American Heart Association has promoted diet and exercise to prevent heart disease, and the American Medical Association (AMA) has been an outspoken opponent against smoking. Professional groups have not been as visible in advocating for patient safety and communicating such concerns to the general public and policy makers. A notable exception has been the formation of the National Patient Safety Foundation (NPSF) by the AMA in 1997 (see Chapter 4). The NSPF has taken a visible role in advocating for improvements in patient safety and communicating with a broad array of audiences. Professional societies can play a role not only in informing their members about patient safety, but also in calling attention to the issue among the general public.

Implementation of activities to increase the role of health professionals in patient safety must occur at multiple levels. Although some professional groups influence and communicate with just their own members, other groups have the potential to influence many audiences. For example, the American Board of Medical Specialties has the potential to influence 24 professional medical societies. The Accreditation Council for Graduate Medical Education and the American Association of Colleges of Nursing have the potential to influence numerous training programs. The Association of American Medical Colleges can influence multiple medical schools and academic medical centers. There are many other similar groups that coordinate across multiple organizations. These "high leverage" groups are critical players in encouraging action among their constituent organizations. They should use their influence to promote greater awareness of patient safety and to consistently reinforce its importance.

STANDARDS FOR DRUGS AND DEVICES

The Food and Drug Administration is a major force in setting standards for medical products and monitoring their safety. FDA regulates prescription and over-the-counter drugs, medical and radiation-emitting devices, and biologics, among other things. This discussion focuses on its activities related to drugs and devices. It should be noted, however, that the FDA regulates manufacturers, not health care organizations or professionals. There are two opportunities for FDA to ensure and enhance patient safety: during its approval process for drugs and devices, and through postmarketing surveillance.

FDA has regulatory authority over the naming, labeling, and packaging of drugs and medical devices. FDA approves a product when it judges that the benefits of using the product outweigh the risks for the intended population and use.[29] For drugs, the approval process examines evidence of the effectiveness of the drug and the safety of the drug when used as intended. For devices, FDA looks at the safety and effectiveness of the device compared to devices already on the market or else looks for reasonable assurance of safety and effectiveness.

A major component of postmarketing surveillance is conducted through adverse event reporting.[30] Reports may be submitted directly to the FDA or through MedWatch, FDA's reporting program. For medical devices, manufacturers are required to report deaths, serious injures, and malfunctions to FDA. User facilities (hospitals, nursing homes) are required to report deaths to both the manufacturer and FDA, and to report serious injuries to the manufacturer. For suspected adverse events associated with drugs, reporting is mandatory for manufacturers and voluntary for physicians, consumers, and others. All reports are entered into the Adverse Event Reporting System (AERS) or another database, which is used to identify problem areas or increased incidence of an event.

FDA receives approximately 235,000 reports annually for adverse drug events and approximately 80,000–85,000 reports on device problems. Despite the extensive testing that FDA requires before drugs and devices are approved, side effects or other problems invariably show up after they have been released and used widely. Not all risks are identified premarketing because study populations in premarketing trials are often too small to detect rare events, studies may not last long enough to detect some events, and study populations may be dissimilar from the general population.[31] Some of these initially unknown risks can be serious or even fatal. The problem is likely to continue and possibly worsen in the future because of the number of new drugs being introduced. In 1998 alone, FDA approved 90 new drugs, 30 new molecular entities (drugs that have never been marketed in this country before), 124 new or expanded uses of already approved drugs, 344 generic drugs, 8 over-the-counter drugs, and 9 orphan drugs, or almost two actions every day of the year.[32] Approximately 48 percent of the prescription drugs on the market today have become available only since 1990.[33] Medications are also the most frequent medical intervention, with an average of 11 prescriptions per person in the United States.[34]

FDA has three general strategies it pursues for corrective action. The first (and most commonly pursued) is negotiation with the manufacturer to make the desired changes. The extent of cooperation from the manufacturers can vary. In terms of drugs, names are the most difficult to change, particularly once a name has been trademarked by the company (Jerry Phillips, OPDRA, personal communication, May 4, 1999). Second, FDA may take regulatory action against manufacturers to require changes. This could include name changes or withdrawal of a product from the market. The final type of action that FDA can take is communication about risks, including letters to physicians, pharmacists, and other health professionals, postings on the Internet, and publication of clinical and consumer journals. FDA decisions about corrective action are made on a case-by-case basis, by considering the unexpectedness and seriousness of the event, the vulnerability of the population affected, and the preventability of the event.[35]

Some concerns have been expressed over the responsiveness of FDA to reported problems. Concerns have related to the timeliness and effectiveness of the agency's response or that the response to a given problem may not be strong enough given its seriousness. For example, five drugs were removed from the market in between September 1997 and September 1998, but almost 20 million people had been exposed to their risks before they were removed.[36] Terfenadine was on the market for 12 years, even though researchers earlier identified it as causing deaths; it was removed from the market by the manufacturer only after a substitute was developed.[37]

There have been calls for better methods for obtaining more information about the harm caused by drugs (e.g., greater use of active surveillance systems that look for indicators of problems rather than waiting for reports to be submitted) or for the establishment of an independent drug safety review board.[38] In the fall of 1998, FDA changed the process for follow-up on reported drug problems with the creation of a new Office of Post-Marketing Drug Risk Assessment (OPDRA). Before, incidents were reviewed by a committee, triaged, and sent back to the division that did the original review. This dispersed responsibility for review and follow-up led to variability in response. Now, OPDRA will conduct an analysis of all reported events and develop recommendations that are sent to the manufacturer and the director of the FDA division that conducted the original review. The division director must report to OPDRA in 60 days on the status of the recommendations. OPDRA estimates that approximately half of the causal factors that contribute to adverse events are issues to which it can respond (e.g., labeling problems); the remainder are outside its scope (e.g., bad handwriting) (Jerry Phillips, OPDRA, personal communication, May 4, 1999).

With regard to medical devices, in recent years, FDA has increased its requirements and guidance to manufacturers on designing devices to take into account human factors principles and user testing. Attention to human factors could improve simplicity of use, standardization of controls, and default to a safe setting during failure (e.g., loss of power). For example, intravenous infusion pumps vary markedly in their mode of operation and types of controls. Because they are expensive, hospitals do not replace old pumps when new ones become available, which results in different models being used. The lack of standardization among the models increases the likelihood of error when the pump is set up. Controls on defibrillators can also vary in position, appearance, and function on different machines, leading to errors when they are used rapidly in emergency situations. Although the increased attention to human factors principles does not affect devices already on the market, over time it is expected that manufacturers will become more accustomed to using human factors in the design of medical devices.

With the passage of the Safe Medical Device Act of 1990, FDA was granted the authority to require manufacturers of medical devices to establish and follow procedures for ensuring that device design addressed the intended use of the device and its users.[39] Final rules for this act became effective in June 1997. FDA has continued to emphasize to manufacturers the importance of human factors and is expected to issue a manual of engineering and design guidelines for manufacturers in 1999.

In terms of drugs, the use of human factors principles could reduce confusion of medications that occur because of brand names that look alike or sound alike, labels that are hard to read, and look-alike packaging. Wrong doses also occur frequently because of factors such as the lack of standardized terms in the display of contents. For example, contents displayed by concentration (e.g., 10 mg/mL) rather than total amount (e.g., 100 mg) can result in an overdose. There may also be inconsistent placement of warnings on a label or inconsistent use of abbreviations. Most recently, more than 100 errors have been reported in the use of Celebrex (prescribed for arthritis) and its confusion with Cerebyx (an antiseizure medication) and Celexa (an antidepressant).[40] FDA does not have guidance for using human factors principles in the packaging, labeling, or naming of drugs as exists relative to medical devices.

SUMMARY

The main sources of standards for health care organizations and professionals today are through licensing and accreditation processes. However, medical errors and patient safety are not an explicit focus of licensing and accreditation. Although licensing and accreditation standards do speak to the characteristics of quality improvement programs, and patient safety and error reduction may be part of these programs, many licensed and fully accredited organizations have yet to implement the most rudimentary systems and processes to ensure patient safety. Furthermore, the extent of variation in licensure within and across states suggests that there is no reliable assurance of safety to patients, even for those facilities and professionals covered under current rules.

Although current standard-setting authorities in health care are not devoting adequate attention to patient safety issues, the committee considered and rejected the option of recommending the creation of yet another regulatory authority. The recommendations contained in this chapter direct the existing regulatory structures to increase attention to patient safety issues. Licensing agencies and accrediting organizations have to hold health care organizations accountable for creating and maintaining safe environments. Professional licensing bodies should consider continuing qualifications over a lifetime of practice, not just at initial licensure. Standards for approving drugs and devices must consider safety for patients in actual use and real-life settings, not just safe production.

The actions of professional groups and group purchasers in setting standards and expectations are also critical. Professional groups shape professional behavior by developing practice guidelines and identifying best practices and through educational, convening and advocacy activities. All could be enhanced by a sharper focus on patient safety issues. Group purchasers have the ability to consider safety issues in their contracting decisions, and to reinforce the importance of safety by providing relevant information to employees and beneficiaries.

REFERENCES

1. Institute of Medicine, *Clinical Practice Guidelines, Directions for a New Program*, eds. Marilyn J. Field and Kathleen N. Lohr, Washington, D.C.: National Academy Press, 1990.

2. "All About OSHA," OSHA 2056 1995 (revised), Occupational Safety and Health Administration, Department of Labor, www.osha.gov.

3. *"Joint Commission Accreditation,"* http://www.jcaho.org/whoweare_frm. html

4. "NCQA Accreditation," *Business and Health*, 17(1):21 (January, 1999).

5. "About URAC," http://www.urac.org

6. General Accounting Office. *Private Health Insurance: Continued Erosion of Coverage Linked to Cost Pressures.* GAO/HEHS 97-122. Washington, DC: July 1997b.

7. Hibbard, Judith H.; Jewett, Jacquelyn J.; Legnini, Mark W., et al. Choosing a Health Plan: Do Large Employers Use the Data. *Health Affairs.* 16(6):172–180, 1997.

8. Washington Business Group on Health and Watson Wyatt Worldwide. *Getting What You Pay for—Purchasing Value in Health Care.* Bethesda, MD: Watson Wyatt Worldwide, 1997.

9. KPMG Peat Marwick. *Health Benefits in 1997.* Montvale, NJ: 1997.

10. http://www.hcfa.gov.

11. "Quality of Care Information, HCFA Contractors, Peer Review Organizations," http://www.hcfa.gov/qlty-56.htm, last updated July 26, 1999.

12. Timothy Cuerdon, Office of Clinical Standards and Quality, Health Care Financing Administration, Testimony to the IOM Subcommittee on Creating an External Environment for Quality, June 15, 1999.

13. "Medicare and Medicaid Survey and Certification," http://www.hcfa.gov/medicaid/scindex.htm

14. O'Neil, Edward H., and the Pew Health Professions Commission, San Francisco, CA: Pew Health Professions Commission, December 1998.

15. Finocchio, Leonard J.; Dower, Catherine M.; Blick, Noelle T., et al., *Strengthen-*

ing *Consumer Protection: Priorities for Health Care Workforce Regulation*, San Francisco, CA; Pew Health Professions Commission, October 1998.

16. *Maintaining State-Based Licensure and Discipline: A Blueprint for Uniform and Effective Regulation of the Medical Profession*, Federation of State Medical Boards of the United States, Inc., 1998. http://www.fsmb.org.

17. Sidney M. Wolfe, "Public Citizen's Health Research Group Ranking of State Medical Boards' Serious Disciplinary Actions in 1998," April, 1999, http://www.citizen. org. Serious disciplinary actions include revocations, surrenders, suspensions and probations/restrictions on licensure.

18. Timberg, Craig, "Virginia's Physician Discipline Board too Slow to Act, Audit Finds," Washington Post, June 15, 1999, p. A20.

19. Finocchio, Dower, Blick, et al., 1998.

20. Finocchio, Dower, Blick, et al., 1998.

21. "What Is ABMS?" http://www.abms.org/purpose.html.

22. Prager, Linda O. Upping the Certification Ante. *American Medical News*. 42(21):1, 1999. Also, American Board of Internal Medicine, *Continuing Professional Development*. September, 1999. See also: Norcini, John J., "Computer-Based Testing Will Soon Be a Reality," *Perspective*, American Board of Internal Medicine, Summer, 1999, p. 3.

23. "A Definition," http://www.ama-assn.org/med-sci/amapsite/about/define.htm.

24. Finocchio, Dower, Blick, et al., 1998.

25. *Computerized Clinical Simulation Testing (CST)*, National Council of State Boards of Nursing, Inc., 1999. http://www.ncsbn.org.

26. Pierce, Ellison C. The 34th Rovenstine Lecture, 40 Years Behind the Mask: Safety Revisited. *Anesthesiology*. 87(4):965–975, 1996.

27. http://www.acc.org/clinical/guidelines.

28. President's Commission on Consumer Protection and Quality in Health Care. *Quality First: Better Health Care for All Americans*. Final Report to the President of the United States, March 1997.

29. Food and Drug Administration, "Managing the Risks From Medical Product Use, Creating a Risk Management Framework," Executive Summary, Report to the FDA Commissioner from the Task Force on Risk Management, May 1999.

30. Additional strategies include field investigations, epidemiological studies and other focused studies.

31. Food and Drug Administration, "Managing the Risks From Medical Product Use, Creating a Risk Management Framework," Report to the FDA Commissioner from the Task Force on Risk Management, U.S. Department of Health and Human Services, May 1999.

32. Food and Drug Administration, "Improving Public Health Through Human Drugs," CDER 1998 Report to the Nation, Center for Drug Evaluation and Research, USDHHS.

33. Shatin, Deborah; Gardner, Jacqueline; Stergachis, Andy; letter. *JAMA*. 281(4): 319–320, 1999.

34. Friedman, Michael A.; Woodcock, Janet; Lumpkin, Murray M., et al. The Safety of Newly Approved Medicines, Do Recent Market Removals Mean There Is a Problem? *JAMA*. 281(18):1728–1934, 1999.

35. Food and Drug Administration. Managing the Risks From Medical Product Use, Creating a Risk Management Framework. Report to the FDA Commissioner from the Task Force on Risk Management, U.S. Department of Health and Human Services, May 1999.

36. Friedman, Woodcock, Lumpkin, et al, 1999. Also Wood, Alastair J.J. The Safety of New Medicines. *JAMA*. 281(18):1753–1754, 1999.

37. Moore, Thomas J; Psaty, Bruce M; Furberg, Curt D. Time to Act on Drug Safety. *JAMA*, 279(19):1571–1573, 1998.

38. Moore, Psaty, and Furberg, 1998. See also Wood, Alastair J.J. and Woosely, Raymond. Making Medicine Safer, The Need for an Independent Drug Safety Review Board. *N Engl J Med*. 339(25):1851–1853, 1998.

39. Weinger, Matthew; Pantiskas, Carl; Wiklund, Michael, et al. Incorporating Human Factors Into the Design of Medical Devices. *JAMA*. 280(17):1484, 1998.

40. Look Alike/Sound Alike Drug Names, Ambiguous or Look-Alike Labeling and Packaging. ISMP Quarterly Action Agenda: April–June, 1999, ISMP Medication Safety Alert, July 14, 1999. Institute for Safe Medication Practices, Pennsylvania.

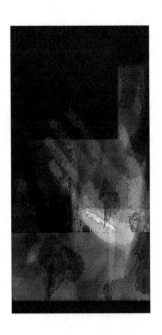

8
Creating Safety Systems in Health Care Organizations

Unsafe acts are like mosquitoes. You can try to swat them one at a time, but there will always be others to take their place. The only effective remedy is to drain the swamps in which they breed. In the case of errors and violations, the "swamps" are equipment designs that promote operator error, bad communications, high workloads, budgetary and commercial pressures, procedures that necessitate their violation in order to get the job done, inadequate organization, missing barriers, and safeguards . . . the list is potentially long but all of these latent factors are, in theory, detectable and correctable before a mishap occurs.[1]

Safety systems in health care organizations seek to prevent harm to patients, their families and friends, health care professionals, contract-service workers, volunteers, and the many other individuals whose activities bring them into a health care setting. Safety is one aspect of quality, where quality includes not only avoiding preventable harm, but also making appropriate care available—providing effective services to those who could benefit from them and not providing ineffective or harmful services.[2]

As defined in Chapter 3, patient safety is *freedom from accidental injury.* This definition and this report intentionally view safety from the perspective of the patient. Accordingly, this chapter focuses specifically on patient safety. The committee believes, however, that a safer environment for patients would also be a safer environment for workers and vice versa, because both are tied to many of the same underlying cultural and systemic issues. As cases in point, hazards to health care workers because of lapses in infection control, fatigue, or faulty equipment may result in injury not only to workers but also to others in the institution.

This chapter introduces what has been learned from other high-risk industries about improving safety. It then discusses key concepts for designing systems and their application in health care. This is followed by a discussion of five principles to guide health care organizations in designing and implementing patient safety programs. Lastly, the chapter discusses a critical area of safety, namely medication safety and illustrates the principles with strategies that health care organizations can use to improve medication safety.

RECOMMENDATIONS

The committee is convinced that there are numerous actions based on both good evidence and principles of safe design that health care organizations can take now or as soon as possible to substantially improve patient safety. Specifically, the committee makes two overarching recommendations: the first concerns leadership and the creation of safety systems in health care settings; the second concerns the implementation of known medication safety practices.

> **RECOMMENDATION 8.1 Health care organizations and the professionals affiliated with them should make continually improved patient safety a declared and serious aim by establishing patient safety programs with a defined executive responsibility. Patient safety programs should: (1) provide strong, clear, and visible attention to safety; implement nonpunitive systems for reporting and analyzing errors within their organizations; (2) incorporate well-understood safety principles, such as, standardizing and simplifying equipment, supplies, and processes; and (3) establish interdisciplinary team training programs, such as simulation, that incorporate proven methods of team management.**

Chief executive officers and boards of trustees must make a serious and ongoing commitment to creating safe systems of care. Other high-risk industries have found that improvements in safety do not occur unless there is commitment by top management and an overt, clearly defined, and continuing effort on the part of all personnel and managers. Like any other program, a meaningful safety program should include senior-level leadership, defined program objectives, plans, personnel, and budget, and should be monitored by regular progress reports to the executive committee and board of directors.

According to Cook,[3] *Safety is a characteristic of systems and not of their components. Safety is an emergent property of systems.* In order for this property to arise, health care organizations must develop a systems orientation to patient safety, rather than an orientation that finds and attaches blame to individuals. It would be hard to overestimate the underlying, critical importance of developing such a culture of safety to any efforts that are made to reduce error. The most important barrier to improving patient safety is lack of awareness of the extent to which errors occur daily in all health care settings and organizations. This lack of awareness exists because the vast majority of errors are not reported, and they are not reported because personnel fear they will be punished.

Health care organizations should establish nonpunitive environments and systems for reporting errors and accidents within their organizations. Just as important, they should develop and maintain an ongoing process for the discovery, clarification, and incorporation of basic principles and innovations for safe design and should use this knowledge in understanding the reasons for hazardous conditions and ways to reduce these vulnerabilities. To accomplish these tasks requires that health care organizations provide resources to monitor and evaluate errors and to implement methods to reduce them.

Organizations should incorporate well-known design principles in their work environment. For example, standardization and simplification are two fundamental human factors principles that are widely used in safe industries and widely ignored in health care.

They should also establish interdisciplinary team training programs—including the use of simulation for trainees and experienced practitioners for personnel in areas such as the emergency department, intensive care unit, and operating room; and incorporating proven methods of managing work in teams as exemplified in aviation (where it is known as crew resource management).

RECOMMENDATION 8.2 Health care organizations should implement proven medication safety practices.

A number of practices have been shown to reduce errors in the medication process and to exemplify known methods for improving safety. The committee believes they warrant strong consideration by health care organizations including hospitals, long-term-care facilities, ambulatory settings, and other health care delivery sites, as well as outpatient and community pharmacies. These methods include: reducing reliance on memory; simplification; standardization; use of constraints and forcing functions; the wise use of protocols and checklists; decreasing reliance on vigilance, handoffs, and multiple data entry; and differentiating among products to eliminate look-alike and sound-alike products.

INTRODUCTION

Errors occur in all industries. Some industrial accidents involve one or a few workers. Others affect entire local populations or ecosystems. In health care, events are well publicized when they appear to be particularly egregious—for example, wrong-site surgery or the death of a patient during what is thought to be a routine, low-risk procedure. Generally, however, accidents are not well publicized; indeed, they may not be known even to the patient or to the family. Because the adverse effects may be separated in time or space from the occurrence, they may not even be recognized by the health care workers involved in the patient's care.

Nevertheless, we know that errors are ubiquitous in all health care settings.[4] Harms range from high-visibility cases to those that are minimal but require additional treatment and time for the patient to recuperate or result in a patient's failure to receive the benefit of appropriate therapy. In aggregate, they represent a huge burden of harm and cost to the American people as described in Chapter 2.

To date, however, those involved in health care management and delivery have not had specific, clear, high-level incentives to apply what has been learned in other industries about ways to prevent error and reduce harm. Consequently, the development of safety systems, broadly understood, has not been a serious and widely adopted priority within health care organizations. This report calls on organizations and on individual practitioners to address patient safety.

Health care is composed of a large set of interacting systems—paramedic, emergency, ambulatory, inpatient care, and home health care; testing and imaging laboratories; pharmacies; and so forth—that are connected in loosely coupled but intricate networks of individuals, teams, procedures, regulations, communications, equipment, and devices that function with diffused management in a variable and uncertain environment.[5] Physicians in community practice may be so tenuously connected that they do not even view themselves as part of a system of care. They may see the hospitals in which they are attendings as platforms for their work. In these and many other ways, the distinct cultures of medicine (and other health professions) add to the idiosyncrasy of health care among high-risk industries.

Nevertheless, experience in other high-risk industries has provided well-understood illustrations that can be used in improving health care safety. Studies of actual accidents, incident-reporting systems, and research on human factors (i.e., the interface of human beings and machines and their performance in complex working environments) have contributed to our growing understanding about how to prevent, detect, and recover from accidents. This has occurred because, despite their differences from health care, all systems have common characteristics that include the use of technologies, the users of these technologies, and an interface between the users and the technologies.[6] The users of technology bring certain characteristics to a task such as the quality of their knowledge and training, level of fatigue, and careful or careless habits. They also bring characteristics that are common to everyone, including difficulty recalling material and making occasional errors.

Safety Systems in High-Risk Industries

The experience in three high-risk industries—chemical and material manufacturing and defense—provides examples of the information and systems that can contribute to improved safety and of the safety achievements that are possible. Claims that health care is unique and therefore not susceptible to a transfer of learning from other industries are not supportable. Rather, the experiences of other industries provide invaluable insight about how to begin the process of improving the safety of health care by learning how to prevent, detect, recover, and learn from accidents.

E.I. du Pont de Nemours and Company

E.I. du Pont de Nemours and Company has one of the lowest rates of occupational injury of any company, substantiation of an 11-point safety philosophy that includes the tenets that all injuries are preventable; that management is responsible and accountable for preventing injury; that safety must be integrated as a core business and personal value; and that deficiencies must be corrected promptly. In 1994, Conoco Refining, a subsidiary, reported only 1.92 work-loss days per 200,000 hours of exposure. In 1998, this rate was further reduced to 0.39. Some of DuPont's plants with more than 2,000 employees have operated for more than 10 years without a lost-time injury, and one plant producing glycolic acid celebrated 50 years without a lost workday.[7] DuPont credits its safety record, at least in part, to its implementation of a nonpunitive system to encourage employees to report near-miss incidents without fear of sanctions or disciplinary measures and its objective to create an *all-pervasive, ever-present awareness of the need to do things safely.*[8,9]

Alcoa, Inc.

Another industry example is Alcoa, which is involved in mining, refining, smelting, fabricating, and recycling aluminum and other materials. Alcoa uses a worldwide on-line safety data system to track incidents, analyze their causes, and share preventive actions throughout all of its holdings. One of its principles is that all incidents, including illnesses, injuries, spills, and excursions, can be prevented whether they are immediate, latent, or cumulative. Although Alcoa reduced its international lost work day rate per 200,000 hours worked from 1.87 in 1987 to 0.42 in 1997, it has recently gone even further and announced a plan to eliminate fatalities and reduce the average injury rate by 50 percent by the end of the year 2000.[10]

Several aspects of these two examples are striking. In comparison to the health care industry, DuPont, Alcoa, and others systematically collect and analyze data about accidents. They have been tracking their own performance over time and are able to compare themselves to others in their industries. They are willing to publish their results as information to which stockholders and employees are entitled and as a source of pride, and their efforts have achieved extremely low and continuously decreasing levels of injury. The importance of a strong culture of safety, as nurtured by both DuPont and Alcoa, is viewed by many in the safety field as being the most critical underlying feature of their accomplishments.

U.S. Navy: Aircraft Carriers

People are quick to point out that health care is very different from a manufacturing process, mostly because of the huge variability in patients and circumstances, the need to adapt processes quickly, the rapidly changing knowledge base, and the importance of highly trained professionals who must use expert judgment in dynamic settings. Though not a biological system, the performance of crews and flight personnel on aircraft carriers provides an example that has features that are closer to those in health care environments than manufacturing.

On an aircraft carrier, fueling aircraft and loading munitions are examples of the risks posed when performing incompatible activities in close proximity. On the flight deck, 100 to 200 people fuel, load munitions, and maintain aircraft that take off and are recovered at 48- to 60-second intervals. The ability to keep these activities separate requires considerable organizational skill and extensive ongoing training to avoid serious injury to flight and nonflight personnel, the aircraft, and the ship. Despite extremely dangerous working conditions and restricted space, the Navy's "crunch rate" aboard aircraft carriers in 1989 was only 1 per 8,000 moves which makes it a very highly reliable, but complex, social organization.*

Students of accident theory emphasize how the interactive complexity of an organization using hazardous technologies seems to defy efforts of system designers and operators to prevent accidents and ensure reliability. In part, this is because individuals are fallible and in part because unlikely and rare (and thus unanticipated) failures in one area are linked in complex systems and may have surprising effects in other systems—the tighter the "coupling," generally, the more likely that failure in one part will affect the reliability of the whole system. Nevertheless, even in such systems, great consistency is achievable using four strategies in particular: the prioritization of safety as a goal; high levels of redundancy, the development of a safety culture that involves continuous operational training, and high-level organizational learning.[11]

Weick and Roberts[12] have studied peacetime flight operations on aircraft carriers as an example of organizational performance requiring nearly continuous operational reliability despite complex patterns of interrelated activities among many people. These activities cannot be fully mapped out beforehand because of changes in weather (e.g., wind direction and strength), sea conditions, time of day and visibility, returning aircraft arrivals, and so forth. Yet, surprisingly, generally mapped out sequences can be carried out with very high reliability in novel situations using improvisation and adaptation and personnel who are highly trained but not highly educated.

---

*A crunch occurs when two aircraft touch while being moved, either on the flight or hangar deck, even if damage is averted.

Naval commanders stress the high priority of safety. They understand the importance of a safety culture and use redundancy (both technical and personnel) and continuous training to prepare for the unexpected. The Navy also understands the need for direct communication and adaptability. Because errors can arise from a lack of direct communication, the ship's control tower communicates directly with each division over multiple channels.

As in health care, it is not possible in such dynamic settings to anticipate and write a rule for every circumstance. Once-rigid orders that prescribed how to perform each operation have been replaced by more flexible, less hierarchical methods. For example, although the captain's commands usually take precedence, junior officers can, and do, change these priorities when they believe that following an order will risk the crew's safety. Such an example demonstrates that even in technologically sophisticated, hazardous, and unpredictable environments it is possible to foster real-time problem solving and to institute safety systems that incorporate a knowledge of human factors.

In summary, efforts such as those described in the three examples have resulted neither in stifled innovation nor loss of competitive benefit; nor have they resulted in unmanageable legal consequences. Rather, they are a source of corporate and employee pride. Characteristics that distinguish successful efforts in other industries include the ability to collect data on errors and incidents within the organization in order to identify opportunities for improvement and to track progress. The companies make these data available to outsiders. Other notable features of these efforts include the importance of leadership and the development of a safety culture, the use of sophisticated methods for the analysis of complex processes, and a striving for balance among standardization where appropriate, yet giving individuals the freedom to solve problems creatively.

KEY SAFETY DESIGN CONCEPTS

Designing safe systems requires an understanding of the sources of errors and how to use safety design concepts to minimize these errors or allow detection before harm occurs. This field is described in greater detail in Chapter 3 which includes an error taxonomy first proposed by Rasmussen[13] and elaborated by Reason[14] to distinguish among errors arising from (1) skill-based slips and lapses; (2) rule-based errors; and (3) knowledge-based mistakes.

Leape has simplified this taxonomy to describe what he calls "the pathophysiology of error." He differentiates between the cognitive mechanisms used when people are engaging in well-known, oft-repeated processes and their cognitive processes when problem solving. The former are handled rapidly, effortlessly, in parallel with other tasks, and with little direct attention. Errors may occur because of interruptions, fatigue, time pressure, anger, anxiety, fear, or boredom. Errors of this sort are expectable, but conditions of work can make them less likely. For example, work activities should not rely on weak aspects of human cognition such as short-term memory. Safe design, therefore, avoids reliance on memory.

Problem-solving processes, by contrast, are slower, are done sequentially (rather than in parallel with other tasks), are perceived as more difficult, and require conscious attention. Errors are due to misinterpretation of the problem that must be solved, lack of knowledge to bring to bear, and habits of thought that cause us to see what we expect to see. Attention to safe design includes simplification of processes so that users who are unfamiliar with them can understand quickly how to proceed, training that simulates problems, and practice in recovery from these problems.

As described in Chapter 3, instances of patient harm are usually attributed to individuals "at the sharp end" who make the visible error. Their prevention, however, requires systems that are designed for safety—that is, systems in which the sources of human error have been systematically recognized and minimized.[15,16]

In recent years, students of system design have looked for ways to avoid error using what has been called by Donald Norman[17] "user-centered design." This chapter draws on six strategies that Norman outlines. They are directed at the design of individual devices so that they can be used reliably and safely for their intended purposes. Although these strategies are aimed at the human–machine interface, they can also be usefully applied to processes of care.

The first strategy is to make things visible—including the conceptual model of the system—so that the user can determine what actions are possible at any moment—for example, how to turn off a piece of equipment, how to change settings, and what is likely to happen if a step in a process is skipped. The second strategy is to simplify the structure of tasks so as to minimize the load on working memory, planning, or problem solving.

A third strategy is what Norman calls the use of *affordances* and *natural mappings*. An affordance is a characteristic of equipment or workspace that communicates how it is to be used, such as a push bar on an outward opening door that indicates where to push. Another example is a telephone handset that is uncomfortable to hold in any position but the correct one.

Natural mapping refers to the relationship between a control and its movement; for example, in steering a car to the right, one turns the wheel right. Natural mapping takes advantage of physical analogies and cultural knowledge to help users understand how to control devices. Other examples of natural mapping are arranging light switches in the same pattern as lights in a lecture room; arranging knobs to match the arrangement of burners on a stove; or using louder sound, an increasingly brighter indicator light, or a wedge shape to indicate a greater amount.

A fourth important strategy is the use of constraints or "forcing functions" to guide the user to the next appropriate action or decision. A constraint makes it hard to do the wrong thing; a forcing function makes it impossible. A classic example of a forcing function is that one cannot start a car that is in gear.

Norman's fifth strategy is to assume that errors will occur and to design and plan for recovery by making it easy to reverse operations and hard to carry out nonreversible ones. An example is the Windows® computer operating system that asks if the user really intends to delete a file, and if so, puts it in a "recycle" folder so that it can still be retrieved.

Finally, Norman advises that if applying the earlier strategies does not achieve the desired results, designers should standardize actions, outcomes, layouts, and displays. An example of standardization is the use of protocols for chemotherapy. An example of simplification is reducing the number of dose strengths of morphine in stock.

Safety systems can be both local and organization wide. Local systems are implemented at the level of a small work group—a department, a unit, or a team of health care practitioners. Such local safety systems should be supported by, and consistent with, organization-wide safety systems.

Anesthesiology is an example of a local, but complex, high-risk, dynamic patient care system in which there has been notably reduced error. Responding to rising malpractice premiums in the mid-1980s, anesthesiologists confronted the safety issues presented by the need for continuing vigilance during long operations but punctuated by the need for rapid problem evaluation and action. They were faced with a heterogeneity of design in anesthesia devices; fatigue and sleep deprivation; and competing institutional, professional, and patient care priorities. By a combination of technological advances (most notably the pulse oximeter), standardization of equipment, and changes in training, they were able to bring about major, sustained, widespread reduction in morbidity and mortality attributable to the administration of anesthesia.[18]

Organization-wide systems, on the other hand, are implemented and monitored at the level of a health care organization. These include programs and processes that cross departmental lines and units. In hospitals, infection control and medication administration are examples of organization-wide systems that encompass externally imposed regulations, institutional policies and procedures, and the actions of individuals who must provide potentially toxic materials at the right time to the right patient.

PRINCIPLES FOR THE DESIGN OF SAFETY SYSTEMS IN HEALTH CARE ORGANIZATIONS

Hospitals and other institutions have long-standing efforts to ensure patient safety in a variety of areas. Appendix E provides an overview of some of these efforts in hospitals. Some have been very effective in certain units or certain hospitals. These activities have not, however, succeeded in eliminating error or injury, and they have not been part of national or even institution-wide, high-priority efforts.

Compared to hospital care, out-of-hospital care—whether in institutions, homes, medical offices or other settings, both the knowledge of the kind and magnitude of errors and the development of safety systems are rudimentary. Safety tends to be addressed narrowly by reliance on education and training, policies, and procedures. There are undoubtedly many reasons for the lack of attention to safety including: small staff size, lack of technical knowledge of effective ways to improve quality or an infrastructure to support deploying this knowledge; lack of recognition of error (because the harm is removed in time or space from the error and because individuals are unharmed); lack of data systems to track and learn from error (most of the adverse drug events studies use emergency visits or hospital admissions to establish a denominator); the speed of change and the introduction of new technologies; and clearly, the same cultural barriers that exist in hospitals—namely, the high premium placed on medical autonomy and perfection and a historical lack of interprofessional cooperation and effective communication.

With the rise in outpatient and office-based surgery, attention is turning to anesthesia safety in settings such as private physician offices, dental, and podiatry offices. For example, guidelines for patient assessment, sedation, monitoring, personnel, emergency care, discharge evaluation, maintenance of equipment, infection control, and the like have been developed by an ad hoc committee for New York State practitioners.[19]

After reviewing what has been learned from other high-risk industries as well as the evidence of practices that can improve health care safety, the committee has identified a set of five principles that it believes can be usefully applied to the design of safe health care, whether in a small group practice, a hospital, or a large health care system. These principles include: (1) providing leadership; (2) respect for human limits in the design process; (3) promoting effective team functioning; (4) anticipating the unexpected; and (5) creating a learning environment.

Principle 1. Provide Leadership

- Make patient safety a priority corporate objective.
- Make patient safety everyone's responsibility.
- Make clear assignments for and expectation of safety oversight.
- Provide human and financial resources for error analysis and systems redesign.
- Develop effective mechanisms for identifying and dealing with unsafe practitioners.

Make Patient Safety a Priority Corporate Objective

The health care organization must develop a culture of safety such that an organization's design processes and workforce are focused on a clear goal—dramatic improvement in the reliability and safety of the care process. The committee believes safety must be an explicit organizational goal that is demonstrated by clear organizational leadership and professional support as seen by the involvement of governing boards, management, and clinical leadership. This process begins when boards of directors demonstrate their commitment to this objective by regular, close oversight of the safety of the institutions they shepherd.

Reviews of progress in reaching goals and system design should be repeated, detailed, quantitative, and demanding. Ways to implement this at the executive level include frequent reports highlighting safety improvement and staff involvement, regular reviews of safety systems, "walk-throughs" to evaluate hazardous areas and designs, incorporation of safety improvement goals into annual business plans, and providing support for sensible forms of simplification.

Recommendations 5.1 and 7.1 also address institutional accountability for safety. Recommendation 5.1 calls for mandatory reporting of serious adverse events by health care organizations. Recommendation 7.1 urges regulators to focus greater attention on patient safety by requiring health care organizations to implement meaningful patient safety programs with defined executive responsibility and for public and private purchasers to provide incentives to health care organizations to demonstrate continuous improvement in patient safety.

Make Patient Safety Everyone's Responsibility

Messages about safety must signal that it is a serious priority of the institution, that there will be increased analysis of system issues with awareness of their complexity, and that they are endorsed by nonpunitive solutions encouraging the involvement of the entire staff. The messages must be well conceived, repeated, and consistent across health care systems, and should stress that safety problems are quality problems. Establishing and clearly conveying such aims are essential in creating safety systems.

All organizations must allocate resources to both production and safety. Although compatible in the long run, they may not be in the short run, which often results in considerable short-run tension. Health care institutions must be both accountable to the public for safety and able to address error and improve their performance without unreasonable fear of the threat of civil liability. This, too, creates tension between ensuring the transparency that allows institutions to be viewed publicly as trustworthy and the confidence that their workers have in identifying and addressing error without fear of formal or informal reprisal.

The committee recommends that health care professionals as well as health care organizations make safety a specific aim. Many, if not most, physicians in community practice view organizations such as hospitals primarily as platforms for their work and do not see themselves as being part of these larger organizations. Nevertheless, their participation in the safety efforts of these organizations is crucial. Health care practitioners should seek to affiliate themselves with organizations that embrace such aims, whether the organizations are hospitals, managed care organizations, medical societies, medical practice groups, or other entities. Rather than treating each error and hazard as a unique, surprising, separate, and sometimes tragic event, they should view the entire organization as a safety system and the search for improved safety and its associated design principles as a lifelong, shared journey.[20] Health professionals should also participate in new efforts that may be undertaken by groups such as a medical practice and the professional groups to which they belong.

Make Clear Assignments and Set Expectations for Safety

Health care organizations should establish meaningful patient safety programs with defined executive responsibility that supports strong, clear, visible attention to safety. Most hospitals have safety programs for workers as required by Occupational Safety and Health Administration (OSHA), but few have patient safety programs. The committee emphasizes that by health care organizations, it intends such safety programs to be established not only by hospitals, but also by other organizations, including managed care organizations and the delivery sites with which they contract. Other industries have found that improvements in safety do not occur unless there are both a commitment by top management and an overt, clearly defined, and continuing effort on the part of all personnel, workers, and managers. As with any other program, a meaningful safety program should include senior-level leadership, defined program objectives, and plans; personnel; budget; collecting and analyzing data; and monitoring by regular progress reports to the executive committee and board of directors. Although safety can never be delegated, there should be clear accountability for safety, a budget, a defined program, and regular reporting to the board.

Provide Human and Financial Resources for Error Analysis and Systems Redesign

Responsibility for management and improvement in risky systems (e.g., medication) as a whole should be clearly located in individuals or cross-functional, cross-departmental teams given the time to discharge this duty. For example, individuals or departments "own" pieces of the medication system, but as a rule, no one manages the medication system as a whole. Oversight of a hospital's medication system as a whole, including its safety and improvement, might be placed under a single clinician, with 50 percent or more of his or her time devoted to this role.

In managed care organizations, quality improvement activities, whether or not developed by accreditation bodies, should focus on patient safety activities and an expectation of major improvements in safety. Although data from ambulatory settings are very limited, the committee believes that such improvement could be on the order of a 50 percent reduction in errors in hospital environments and could be greatly reduced in outpatient settings.

Develop Effective Mechanisms for Identifying and Dealing with Unsafe Practitioners

Although almost all accidents result from human error, it is now recognized that these errors are usually induced by faulty systems that "set people up" to fail. Correction of these systems failures is the key to safe performance of individuals. Systems design—how an organization works, its processes and procedures—is an institutional responsibility. Only the institution can redesign its systems for safety; the great majority of effort in improving safety should focus on safe systems, and the health care organization itself should be held responsible for safety.

The committee recognizes, however, that some individuals may be incompetent, impaired, uncaring, or may even have criminal intent. The public needs dependable assurance that such individuals will be dealt with effectively and prevented from harming patients. Although these represent a small proportion of health care workers, they are unlikely to be amenable to the kinds of approaches described in detail in this chapter. Registration boards and licensure discipline is appropriately reserved for those rare individuals identified by organizations as a threat to patient safety, whom organizations are already required by state law to report.

Historically, the health system has not had effective ways of dealing with dangerous, reckless, or incompetent individuals and ensuring they do not harm patients. Although the health professions have a long history of work in this area, current systems do not, as a whole, work reliably or promptly. The lack of timeliness has been a special problem. Numerous reasons have been advanced for the lack of more timely and effective response by professions and institutions. Requirements posed by legal due process can be very slow and uncertain; the need for, but difficulty in arranging, excellent supervision has stymied efforts at retraining; and matching individual needs to adult learning principles and retraining that is tailored to specific deficits has been problematic. With this acknowledged, the committee believes that health care organizations should use and rely on proficiency-based credentialing and privileging to identify, retrain, remove, or redirect physicians, nurses, pharmacists, or others who cannot competently perform their responsibilities. With effective safety systems in place, the committee believes it will be easier for those within organizations to identify and act on information about such individuals. If these systems are working properly, unsafe professionals will be identified and dealt with *before* they cause serious patient injury.

Principle 2. Respect Human Limits in Process Design

- Design jobs for safety.
- Avoid reliance on memory.
- Use constraints and forcing functions.
- Avoid reliance on vigilance.
- Simplify key processes.
- Standardize work processes.

Human beings have many intellectual strengths, such as their large memory capacity; a large repertory of responses; flexibility in applying these responses to information inputs; and an ability to react creatively and effectively to the unexpected. However, human beings also have well-known limitations, including difficulty in attending carefully to several things at once, difficulty in recalling detailed information quickly, and generally poor computational ability.[21] Respecting human abilities involves recognizing the strengths of human beings as problem solvers, but minimizing reliance on weaker traits. Several strategies are particularly important when considering such human factors: designing jobs for safety; avoiding reliance on memory and vigilance; using constraints and forcing functions; and simplifying and standardizing key processes.

Design Jobs for Safety

Designing jobs with attention to human factors means attending to the effect of work hours, workloads, staffing ratios, sources of distraction, and an inversion in assigned shifts (which affects worker's circadian rhythms) and their relationship to fatigue, alertness, and sleep deprivation. Designing jobs to minimize distraction may, for example, mean setting aside times, places, or personnel for specific tasks such as calculating doses or mixing intravenous solutions. Designing jobs for safety also means addressing staff training needs and anticipating harm that may accompany downsizing, staff turnover, and the use of part-time workers and "floats" who may be unfamiliar with equipment and processes in a given patient care unit. To the extent that these barriers presented by departmental affiliation and disciplinary training prevent caregivers from working cooperatively and developing new safety systems, job design requires attention not only to the work of the individual but also to the work and training of multidisciplinary teams.

Avoid Reliance on Memory

Health care organizations should use protocols and checklists wisely and whenever appropriate. Examples of the sensible design and use of protocols and checklists are to ensure their routine updating and constructing checklists so that the usual state is answered as yes. Protocols for the use of heparin and insulin, for example, have been developed by many hospitals.[22] An Institute of Medicine report on the development of clinical guidelines suggests features for assessing guidelines that address their substance and process of development. Examples of attributes concerning the substance of guidelines are their validity and clinical applicability. Examples of the process of development include its clarity and documentation of the strength of the evidence.[23]

For medications, ways to reduce reliance on memory are the use of drug–drug interaction checking software and dosing cards (e.g., laminated cards that can be posted at nursing stations or carried in the pocket) that include standard order times, doses of antibiotics, formulas for calculating pediatric doses, and common chemotherapy protocols.[24]

Caution about using protocols wisely derives from the need to generalize and simplify, but to recognize that not all steps of a protocol may be appropriate. Rapid increases in knowledge and changing technology mean that a system for regular updating of protocols should be built into their production.

Use Constraints and Forcing Functions

Constraints and forcing functions are employed to guide the user to the next appropriate action or decision and to structure critical tasks so that errors cannot be made. They are important in designing defaults for devices and for processes such as diagnostic and therapeutic ordering. When a device fails, it should always default to the safest mode; for example, an infusion pump should default to shutoff, rather than free flow.

Examples of the use of constraints in ordering medications are pharmacy computers that will not fill an order unless allergy information, patient weight, and patient height are entered. Another forcing function is the use of special luer locks for syringes and indwelling lines that have to be matched before fluid can be infused. Removal of concentrated potassium chloride from patient floor stock is a (negative) forcing function.[25] Less restrictive, but user-oriented approaches to design are the use of affordances and natural mappings.

Avoid Reliance on Vigilance

Human factors research has taught us that individuals cannot remain vigilant for long periods during which little happens that requires their action, and it is unreasonable to expect them to do so. Health care has many examples of automation used to reduce reliance on vigilance: using robotic dispensing systems in the pharmacy and infusion pumps that regulate the flow of intravenous fluids. Although automation is intended to reduce the need for vigilance, there are also pitfalls in relying on automation if a user learns to ignore alarms that are often wrong or becomes inattentive or inexpert in a given process, or if the effects of errors remain invisible until it is too late to correct them. Well-designed pumps give information about the reason for an alarm, have moderate sensitivity, and prevent free flow when the unit is turned off or fails.

Other approaches for accommodating the need for vigilance have been developed. These include providing checklists and requiring their use at regular intervals, limiting long shifts, and rotating staff who must perform repetitive functions.[26]

Simplify Key Processes

Simplifying key processes can minimize problem solving and greatly reduce the likelihood of error. Simplifying includes reducing the number of handoffs required for a process to be completed (e.g., decreasing multiple order and data entry). Examples of processes that can usually be simplified are: writing an order, then transcribing and entering it in a computer, or having several people record and enter the same data in different databases. Other examples of simplification include limiting the choice of drugs available in the pharmacy, limiting the number of dose strengths, maintaining an inventory of frequently prepared drugs, reducing the number of times per day a drug is administered, keeping a single medication administration record, automating dispensing, and purchasing easy-to-use and maintain equipment.[27]

Standardize Work Processes

Standardization reduces reliance on memory. It also allows newcomers who are unfamiliar with a given process or device to use it safely. In general, standardizing device displays (e.g., readout units), operations (e.g., location of the on–off switch), and doses is important to reduce the likelihood of error. Examples of standardizing include not stocking look-alike products; the use of standard order forms, administration times, prescribing conventions; protocols for complex medication administration; reducing the numbers of available dose strengths and the times of drug administration, placement of supplies and medications; and types of equipment.[28]

Sometimes devices or medications cannot be standardized. When variation is unavoidable, the principle followed should be to differentiate clearly. An example is to identify look-alike, but different, strengths of a narcotic by labeling the higher concentration with bright orange tape.

Principle 3. Promote Effective Team Functioning

- Train in teams those who are expected to work in teams.
- Include the patient in safety design and the process of care.

Train in Teams Those Who Are Expected to Work in Teams

People work together in small groups throughout health care, whether in a multispecialty group practice, in interdisciplinary teams assembled for the care of a specific clinical condition (e.g., teams that care for children with congenital problems, oncology teams, end-of-life care), in operating rooms, and in ICUs. However, members of the team are typically trained in separate disciplines and educational programs. They may not appreciate each other's strengths or recognize weaknesses except in crises, and they may not have been trained together to use new or well-established technologies.

The committee believes that health care organizations should establish team training programs for personnel in critical care areas (e.g., the emergency department, intensive care unit, operating room) using proven methods such as the crew resource management techniques employed in aviation, including simulation. People make fewer errors when they work in teams. When processes are planned and standardized, each member knows his or her responsibilities as well as those of teammates, and members "look out" for one another, noticing errors before they cause an accident. In an effective interdisciplinary team, members come to trust one another's judgments and attend to one another's safety concerns.

The risk associated with a move to adopt such training from fields such as aviation is in borrowing these training technologies too literally. Although the team issues associated with performance in aviation and medicine have strong parallels in medical settings, effective training must be based not on adopting the training technologies too literally but on adapting them to the practices and personnel in the new setting.

Include the Patient in Safety Design and the Process of Care

The members of a team are more than the health care practitioners. A team includes the practitioners, patients, and technologies used for the care of these patients. Whenever possible, patients should be a part of the care process. This includes attention to their preferences and values, their own knowledge of their condition, and the kinds of treatments (including medications) they are receiving. Patients should also have information about the technologies that are used in their care, whether for testing, as an adjunct to therapy, or to provide patient information. Examples of ways to share such information with patients include reviewing with patients a list of their medications, doses, and times to take them; how long to take them; and precautions about interactions with alternative therapies or with alcohol, possible side effects, and any activities that should be avoided such as driving or the use of machinery. Patients should also receive a clearly written list of their medications and instructions for use that they can keep and share with other clinicians.[29]

Principle 4. Anticipate the Unexpected

- Adopt a proactive approach: examine processes of care for threats to safety and redesign them before accidents occur.
- Design for recovery.
- Improve access to accurate, timely information.

Adopt a Proactive Approach: Examine Processes of Care for Threats to Safety and Redesign Them Before Accidents Occur

Technology is ubiquitous in acute care, long-term care, ambulatory surgical centers, and home care. The value of automating repetitive, time-consuming, and error-prone tasks has long been understood and embraced in health care. The increasing use of technologies goes well beyond bedside or operating room devices. It includes emerging technologies that range from molecular, cellular, genetic, and pharmaceutical interventions; to patient-administered technologies (e.g., prescribed medications, monitors, patient-controlled analgesia); to robotic and remote technologies such as remote ICU and telemedicine, Internet-based systems, and expert systems.[30-33]

At the same time, the human–machine interface is a focus of much preventive effort. Indeed, many technologies are engineered not only for safe operation in the care process, but specifically for the purpose of preventing error. Such technologies include automated order entry systems; pharmacy software to alert about drug interactions; and decision support systems such as reminders, alerts, and expert systems.

Health care organizations should expect any new technology to introduce new sources of error and should adopt the custom of automating cautiously, alert to the possibility of unintended harm. Despite the best intentions of designers, the committee emphasizes that *ALL technology introduces new errors, even when its sole purpose is to prevent errors.* Therefore as change occurs, health systems should anticipate trouble. Indeed, Cook emphasizes that future failures cannot be forestalled by providing simply another layer of defense against failure.[34] Rather, safe equipment design and use depend on a chain of involvement and commitment that begins with the manufacturer and continues with careful attention to the vulnerabilities of a new device or system. Prevention requires the continuous redesign and implementation of safe systems to make error increasingly less likely, for example:

- using order entry systems that provide real-time alerts if a medication order is out of range for weight or age, or is contraindicated;
- using bar coding for positive identification and detection of misidentified patients, records, and so forth;
- using "hear back" for oral orders and instructions—for example, having a pharmacist repeat a phoned-in prescription to the caller; and
- monitoring vital signs, blood levels, and other laboratory values for patients receiving hazardous drugs.

Double-checking for particularly vulnerable parts of the system is another approach to preventing patient injury. One approach could be the use of tiger teams. The military phrase *tiger team* originated with a group whose purpose is to penetrate security and test security measures. Professional tiger teams are now used to test corporate systems for vulnerability, particularly to hackers. The idea of using teams with sophisticated knowledge of technical systems to test and anticipate the ways health systems can go wrong could well be adopted by health care organizations.

Patient safety, as well as business outcomes, should be anticipated when reorganization, mergers, and other organization-wide changes in staffing, responsibilities, work loads, and relationship among caregivers result in new patterns of care. Such major changes often have safety implications that can be anticipated and tracked.

Design for Recovery

Prevention is one way to reduce error, but once the error rate and the transmission of the error to patients become very small, incremental gains are increasingly difficult to achieve. Another approach is to work on the processes of recovery when an error occurs. Designing for recovery means making errors visible, making it easy to reverse operations and hard to carry out nonreversible ones, duplicating critical functions or equipment as necessary to detect error, and intercepting error before harm occurs. Although errors cannot be reduced to zero, we should strive to reduce to zero the instances in which error harms a patient. A reliable system has procedures and attributes that make errors visible to those working in the system so that they can be corrected before causing harm.

Examples of procedures to mitigate injury are

- keeping antidotes for high-risk drugs up-to-date and easily accessible;
- having procedures in place for responding quickly to adverse events, such that these processes are standardized across units and personnel are provided with drills to familiarize them with the procedures and the actions each person should take;
- equipment that defaults to the least harmful mode in a crisis; and
- simulation training.

Another example of ways to prevent and to mitigate harm is simulation training. Simulation is a training and feedback method in which learners practice tasks and processes in lifelike circumstances using models or virtual reality, with feedback from observers, other team members, and video cameras to assist improvement of skills.[35] Simulation for modeling crisis management (e.g., when a patient goes into anaphylactic shock or a piece of equipment fails) is sometimes called "crew resource management," an analogy with airline cockpit crew simulation.[36-41] Such an approach carries forward the tradition of disaster drills in which organizations have long participated. In such simulation, small groups that work together—whether in the operating room, intensive care unit, or emergency department—learn to respond to a crisis in an efficient, effective, and coordinated manner.

In the case of the operating room (OR) this means attempting to develop simulation that involves all key players (e.g., anesthesia, surgery, nursing) because many problems occur at the interface between disciplines.[42] Although a full OR simulator has been in operation for some years at the University of Basel (Switzerland), the range of surgical procedures that can be simulated is limited. It will be a great challenge to develop simulation technology and simulators that will allow full, interdisciplinary teams to practice interpersonal and technical skills in a non-jeopardy environment where they can receive meaningful feedback and reinforcement.

Improve Access to Accurate, Timely Information

Information about the patient, medications, and other therapies should be available at the point of patient care, whether they are routinely or rarely used. Examples of ways to make such information available are the following

- Have a pharmacist available on nursing units and on rounds.
- Use computerized lab data that alert clinicians to abnormal lab values.
- Place lab reports and medication administration records at the patient's bedside.
- Place protocols in the patient's chart.
- Color-code wristbands to alert of allergies.
- Track errors and near misses and report them regularly.
- Accelerate laboratory turn around time.

Organizations can improve up-to-date access to information about infrequently used drugs by distributing newsletters and drug summary sheets; and ensuring access to Internet-based web sites, the *Physicians Desk Reference*, formularies, and other resources for ordering, dispensing, and administering medications.

Clearly, any discussion of the availability of accurate, timely information for patient care must stress the need for electronic databases and interfaces to allow them to be fully integrated, and the committee underscores the need for data standards and the development of integrated computer-based databases and knowledge servers.

Health care organizations should join other groups in contributing to the development of standardized data sets for patient records. Uniform standards for connectivity, terminology, and data sharing are critical if the creation and maintenance of health care databases are to be efficient and their information is to be accurate and complete. National standards for the protection of data confidentiality are also needed. The committee urges that health care organizations join payers, vendors, quasi-public standard-setting bodies (such as the National Institute of Standards and Technology (NIST) and American National Standards Institute (ANSI)), federal agencies, and advisory groups in working to facilitate standards-setting efforts and otherwise become full participants in the multidisciplinary effort that is now under way.

Despite the computer-based patient record being "almost here" for 45 years, it has still not arrived. Its advantages are clear: computer-based patient records and other systems give physicians and other authorized personnel the ability to access patient data without delay at any time in any place (e.g., in an emergency or when the patient is away from home); ensure that services are obtained and track outcomes of treatment; and aggregate data from large numbers of patients, both to measure outcomes of treatment; and to promptly recognize complications of new drugs, devices, and treatments.[43]

The committee also believes that organizations, individually and in collaboration, must commit to using information technology to manage their knowledge bases and processes of care. Doing so will require the integration of systems that are patient specific, allow population-based analyses, and systems that manage the case process through reminder, decision support, and guidance grounded in evidence-based knowledge.

Principle 5. Create a Learning Environment

- Use simulations whenever possible.
- Encourage reporting of errors and hazardous conditions.
- Ensure no reprisals for reporting of errors.
- Develop a working culture in which communication flows freely regardless of authority gradient.
- Implement mechanisms of feedback and learning from error.

Use Simulations Whenever Possible

As described under Principle 4, health care organizations and teaching institutions should participate in the development and use of simulation for training novice practitioners, problem solving, and crisis management, especially when new and potentially hazardous procedures and equipment are introduced. Crew resource management techniques, combined with simulation, have substantially improved aviation safety and can be modified for health care use. Early successful experience in emergency department and operating room use indicates they should be more widely applied.[44]

As noted, health care—particularly in dynamic setting such as operating rooms and emergency departments—involves tightly coupled systems. For this reason, crew resource management can be very valuable in reducing (though probably not eliminating) error. For such programs to achieve their potential, however, requires a thorough understanding of the nature of team interactions, the etiology and frequency of errors, and the cultures of each organization into which they are introduced.

Encourage Reporting of Errors and Hazardous Conditions

The culture of a health care organization plays a critical role in how well errors are detected and handled. Medical training and the culture instilled during this training have considerable strengths—emphasizing autonomy of action and personal responsibility. It has also led to a culture of hierarchy and authority in decision making and to a belief that mistakes should not be made. If they do occur, mistakes are typically treated as a personal and professional failure.[45] Because medical training is typically isolated from the training of other health professionals, people have not learned to work together to share authority and collaborate in problem solving. Attempting to change such a culture to accept error as normal is difficult, and accepting the occurrence of error as an opportunity to learn and improve safety is perhaps even more difficult. As noted at the beginning of this chapter, it requires at a minimum that members of the organization believe that safety is really a priority in their organization, that reporting will really be nonpunitive, and that improving patient safety requires fixing the system, not fixing blame. It will almost surely require changes in the way health care professionals are trained in terms not only of their own professional work, but also of how they learn to work together.

Ensure No Reprisals for Reporting of Errors

Health care organizations should establish nonpunitive environments and systems for reporting errors and accidents. The most important barrier to improving patient safety is lack of awareness of the extent to which errors occur daily in all health care organizations. It is difficult to remedy problems that you do not know exist. This lack of awareness occurs because in most cases, errors are not reported.

Studies have shown that typically less than five percent of known errors are reported, and many are unknown.[46] When punishment is eliminated, reporting soars.

Important characteristics of reporting systems within organizations include that they be voluntary, have minimal restrictions on acceptable content, include descriptive accounts and stories (i.e., not be a simple checklist), be confidential, and be accessible for contributions from all clinical and administrative staff. Once submitted, they should be de-identified by reporter and analyzed by experts. Finally, staff should be given timely feedback on the results and how problems will be addressed.[47]

Develop a Working Culture in Which Communication Flows Freely Regardless of Authority Gradient

Organizations also have to foster a management style in dealing with error that supports voluntary reporting and analysis of errors so there are no reprisals and no impediments to information flowing freely against a power gradient.

Techniques for such communication can be taught. Military and civilian aviation has taught senior pilots to respect and listen to junior colleagues, and that copilots and junior officers have the responsibility to communicate clearly their concerns about safety. Superiors have the responsibility to reply to these concerns according to the "two-challenge rule." This rule states that if a pilot is clearly challenged twice about an unsafe situation during a flight without a satisfactory reply, the subordinate is empowered to take over the controls. During military briefings and debriefings, attendees are also expected to express their concerns about safety aspects of an operation.

Bringing about such change in communication patterns within the health care environment, particularly in teaching environments, is without question a major undertaking that begins at least with medical residency training and nursing training. For the leaders of health care teams, it requires learning leadership behavior that encourages and expects all members of the team to internalize the need to be alert to threats to patient safety and to feel that their contributions and concerns are respected.

Implement Mechanisms of Feedback and Learning from Error

In order to learn from error, health care organizations will have to establish and maintain environments and systems for analyzing errors and accidents so that the redesign of processes is informed rather than an act of tampering. There are five important phases to improving safety. The first is the reporting of events in sufficiently rich detail to create a "story" about what occurred. The second is understanding the story in order to make its meaning clear. The third is to develop recommendations for improvement. The fourth is implementation, and the fifth is tracking the changes to learn what new safety problems may have been introduced.

Organizations should develop and maintain an ongoing process for the discovery, clarification, and incorporation of basic principles and innovations for safe design, and should use this knowledge to understand the reasons for hazardous conditions and ways to reduce these vulnerabilities. Organizations require sound, scientifically grounded theories about error and safety. They should draw on the health care industry, other industries, and research on human factors and engineering, organizational and social psychology, and cognitive psychology for useful ideas. Analysis of events leading to error should draw on this knowledge base. Organizational expertise may have to be augmented by external technical assistance, especially in small institutions without the resources to support such activities and expertise internally. Such assistance might come from academically based research centers, trade associations, and professional groups.

Research and analysis are not luxuries in the operation of safety systems. They are essential steps in the effective redesign of systems because analysis provides the information needed for effective prevention. As safety research in other fields has taught us, when a major event occurs that results in patient harm or death, both active and latent errors were present. Investigation of active errors has focused on the individuals present and the circumstances immediately surrounding the event. However, such an explanation is often not only premature and uninformed, but it is usually unhelpful in preventing future events. Understanding the latent errors whose adverse consequences may lie dormant within the system requires considerable technical and systems knowledge about technical work and the way organizational factors play out in this technical work. It also requires understanding the roles of resource limitations, conflicts, uncertainty, and complexity.

Two other ways in which organizations can improve their performance through shared learning are by benchmarking and collaboration. Benchmarking is a way to compare oneself or one's organization against the "best in class." While learning about and finding ways to implement the best practices they can identify, organizations can implement sets of practical, time-series measures that can help them learn whether the steps they have taken are improving safety.[48] Organizations can also collaborate with other facilities, even within their market areas, to understand patterns of error and new approaches to prevention. For example, the New England Cardiovascular Project, the Vermont-Oxford Neonatal Network, and multisite research on the organization and delivery of care in intensive care units have demonstrated the gains that are possible from such collaborative work.[49,50]

The committee strongly encourages organizations to participate in voluntary reporting systems. Chapter 5 provides descriptions of some voluntary reporting systems available in the health care industry, and the committee has recommended that voluntary reporting initiatives be encouraged and expanded.

MEDICATION SAFETY

As described in Chapter 2, a good deal of research has identified medication error as a substantial source of preventable error in hospitals. In addition, organizations and researchers have paid considerable attention to methods of preventing such errors, and there is reasonable agreement about useful approaches. For this reason, the remainder of this chapter focuses on medication administration to illustrate how the principles for creating safety systems might be applied, including the need for a systems approach. It focuses on hospitals because most of the research in this area and virtually all the data are hospital-based but recognizes that many of the strategies apply to ambulatory and other settings as well.

Errors increase with complexity. Complexity in the medication system arises from several sources; including the extensive knowledge and information that are necessary to correctly prescribe a medication regimen for a particular patient; the intermingling of medications of varying hazard in the pharmacy, during transport, and on the patient care units; and the multiple tasks performed by nurses, of which medication preparation and administration are but a few. Because the burden of harm to patients is great, the cost to society is large, and knowledge of how to prevent the most common kinds of errors is well known, the committee singles out medication safety as a high priority area for all health care organizations.

A number of practices have been shown to reduce errors in the medication process and should be in place in all hospitals and other health care organizations in which they are appropriate.[51-53]

Selected Strategies to Improve Medication Safety

- Adopt a system-oriented approach to medication error reduction.
- Implement standard processes for medication doses, dose timing, and dose scales in a given patient care unit.
- Standardize prescription writing and prescribing rules.
- Limit the number of different kinds of common equipment.
- Implement physician order entry.
- Use pharmaceutical software.
- Implement unit dosing.
- Have the central pharmacy supply high-risk intravenous medications.
- Use special procedures and written protocols for the use of high-risk medications.
- Do not store concentrated solutions of hazardous medications on patient care units.
- Ensure the availability of pharmaceutical decision support.
- Include a pharmacist during rounds of patient care units.
- Make relevant patient information available at the point of patient care.
- Improve patients' knowledge about their treatment.

Several organizations have recently focused attention on medication safety, and a number have compiled recommendations for safe medication practices, particularly in the inpatient environment. Most recently, these include the National Patient Safety Partnership,[54] the Massachusetts Coalition for the Prevention of Medical Errors (1999),[55] the Institute for Healthcare Improvement (1998),[56] the National Coordinating Council for Medication Error Reporting and Prevention (NCCMERP); and the American Society for Health-System Pharmacists.[57]

As illustrated in Table 8.1, most of the groups' recommendations are consistent with one another. Although each has been implemented by a large number of hospitals, none has been universally adopted, and some are not in

TABLE 8-1 Comparison of Institute of Medicine (IOM) Strategies Regarding Medication Practices and Recommendations from Other Organizations

IOM Strategy	American Society of Health-System Pharmacists	National Coordinating Council for Medication Error Reporting and Prevention
Implement standard processes for medication doses, dose timing, and dose scales in a given patient care unit		
Standardize prescription writing and prescribing rules		All prescription orders should be written using the metric system except for therapies that use standard units. The term "units" should be spelled out. A leading zero should always precede a decimal expression of less than one. Prescribers should avoid use of abbreviations
Limit the number of different kinds of common equipment		
Implement physician order entry	Establish processes in which prescribers enter medication orders directly into computer systems	Prescribers should move to a direct, computerized order entry system
Use pharmaceutical software		
Implement unit dosing	Use unit dose medication distribution and pharmacy-based intravenous medication admixture systems	The medication order should include drug name, exact metric weight or concentration, and dosage form

Institute for Healthcare Improvement	National Patient Safety Partnership	Massachusetts Coalition for the Prevention of Medical Errors
Reduce reliance on memory; simplify; standardize	Standardize drug packaging, labeling, storage	
Differentiate: eliminate look-alikes and sound-alikes	Avoid abbreviations	
Decrease multiple entry	Computerize drug order entry	Implement computerized prescriber order entry systems when technically and financially feasible in light of a hospital's existing resources and technological development.
		Encourage pharmacy system software vendors to incorporate an adequate set of checks into computerized hospital pharmacy systems
	Use "unit dose" drug systems (packaged and labeled in standard patient doses)	Maintain unit-dose distribution systems (either manufacturer prepared or repackaged by pharmacy) for all non-emergency medications.

TABLE 8-1 Continued

IOM Strategy	American Society of Health-System Pharmacists	National Coordinating Council for Medication Error Reporting and Prevention
Central pharmacy should supply high-risk intravenous medications		
Use special procedures and written protocols for the use of high-risk medications		
Do not store concentrated solutions of hazardous medications on patient care units		
Ensure the availability of pharmaceutical decision support	All medication orders before a first dose should be routinely reviewed by a pharmacist and all staff should seek resolution whenever there is a question of safety	
Include a pharmacist during rounds of patient care units	Assign pharmacists to work in patient care areas in direct collaboration with prescribers and those administering medications	

Institute for Healthcare Improvement	National Patient Safety Partnership	Massachusetts Coalition for the Prevention of Medical Errors
	Use pharmacy-based IV and drug mixing programs	Institute pharmacy-based IV admixture systems
Use protocols and checklists wisely	Limit access to high hazard drugs and use protocols for high hazard drugs.	Develop special procedures for high-risk drugs using a multi-disciplinary approach. Including written guidelines, checklists, pre-printed orders, double-checks, special packaging, special labeling, and education
		Remove concentrated potassium chloride (KCl) vials from nursing units and patient care areas. Stock only diluted premixed IV solutions on units.
		Have a pharmacist available on-call after hours of pharmacy operation.
		Information on new drugs, infrequently used drugs, and non-formulary drugs should be made easily accessible to clinicians prior to ordering, dispensing, and administering medications

TABLE 8-1 Continued

IOM Strategy	American Society of Health-System Pharmacists	National Coordinating Council for Medication Error Reporting and Prevention
Make relevant patient information available at the point of patient care	Evaluate the use of machine-readable coding (e.g., bar coding) in their medication-use processes	Prescribers should include the age and when appropriate, the weight of the patient on the prescription or medication order
Adopt a system-oriented approach to medication error reduction	Approach medication errors as system failures and seek system solutions to preventing them	
Improve patient's knowledge about their treatment		Prescription orders should include a brief notation of purpose unless considered inappropriate Prescribers should not use vague instructions such as "Take as directed" as the sole direction for use
	Develop better systems for monitoring and reporting adverse drug events	

Institute for Healthcare Improvement	National Patient Safety Partnership	Massachusetts Coalition for the Prevention of Medical Errors
Improve access to information	Put allergies and medications on patient records Require machine-readable labeling (bar coding)	Consider the use of machine-readable coding (i.e., bar coding) in the medication administration process Encourage the use of computer-generated or electronic medication administration records (MAR)
Increase feedback; train for teamwork; drive out fear; obtain leadership commitment; improve direct communication		Adopt a systems-oriented approach to medication error reduction; promote a non-punitive atmosphere for reporting of errors which values the sharing of information
Improve access to information	Educate patients Patients should tell physicians about all medications they are taking and ask for information in terms they understand before accepting medications	Educate patients in the hospital, at discharge, and in ambulatory settings about the safe and accurate use of their medications
Organize the work environment for safety		

place in even a majority of hospitals. Based on evidence and drawing on the principles described in this chapter, this IOM committee joins other groups in calling for implementation of proven medication safety practices as described below.

Adopt a System-Oriented Approach to Medication Error Reduction

Throughout this chapter, emphasis is put on the development of a system-oriented approach that prevents and identifies errors and minimizes patient harm from errors that do occur. It involves a cycle of anticipating problems, for example with changes in staffing or the introduction of new technologies, adopting the five principles described, tracking and analyzing data as errors and near misses occur, and using those data to modify processes to prevent further occurrences. None of these steps is useful alone. When taken together with strong executive leadership in a nonpunitive environment and with appropriate resources, they become extremely powerful in improving safety.

Implement Standard Processes for Medication Doses, Dose Timing, and Dose Scales in a Given Patient Care Unit

One of the most powerful means of preventing errors of all kinds is to standardize processes. If doses, times, and scales are standardized, it is easier for personnel to remember them, check them, and cross-check teammates who are administering the medications.

Standardize Prescription Writing and Prescribing Rules

A host of common shortcuts in prescribing have frequently been found to cause errors. Abbreviations are the major offender because they can have more than one meaning. Other "traps" include the use of "q" (as in qid, qod, qd, qh), which is easily misread, and the use of the letter "u" for "unit." Failure to specify all of the elements of an order (form, dose, frequency, route) also leads to errors. Putting such information in computerized order entry forms can help eliminate such errors.

Limit the Number of Different Kinds of Common Equipment

Simplification—reducing the number of options—is almost as effective as standardization in reducing medication errors. Just as with limiting medications to one dose decreases the chance of error, limiting the types of equipment (e.g., infusion pumps) available on a single patient care unit will improve safety. Unless all such equipment has the same method of setup and operation, having several different types of infusion pumps and defibrillators increases the likelihood of misuse, sometimes with disastrous consequences.

Implement Physician Order Entry

Having physicians enter and transmit medication orders on-line (computerized physician order entry) is a powerful method for preventing medication errors due to misinterpretation of hand-written orders. It can ensure that the dose, form, and timing are correct and can also check for potential drug–drug or drug–allergy interactions and patient conditions such as renal function. In one before-and-after comparison,[58] nonintercepted serious medication errors decreased by more than half (from 10.7 to 4.86 events per 1,000 patient-days).

Direct order entry reduces errors at all stages of the medication process, not just in prescribing[60] and it has been recommended by National Patient Safety Partnership, a coalition of health care organizations.*

One study estimated cost savings attributable to preventable adverse drug events (ADEs) at more than $4,000 per event. Direct savings from reduction of ADEs were estimated to be more than $500,000 annually at one teaching hospital, with an overall savings from all decision support interventions related to order entry of between $5 to 10 million per year.[61] A computerized system costing $1 to 2 million could pay for itself in three to five years, while preventing injury to hundreds of patients each year.

Until computerized order entry is implemented, much of the safety benefit may be realized by manual systems that use standard order forms for highly prevalent circumstances, (e.g., myocardial infarction, use of heparin) if the forms are used as completed by clinicians and not transcribed.

Computerized order entry can be a valuable safety adjunct for laboratory and radiology ordering as well as for medication and to achieve the

---

*Member organizations include the American Hospital Association, American Medical Association, American Nurses Association, Association of American Medical Colleges, Agency for Healthcare Research and Quality, Food and Drug Administration, Health Care Financing Administration, Joint Commission on the Accreditation of Healthcare Organizations, Institute for Healthcare Improvement, National Institute for Occupational Safety and Health, National Patient Safety Foundation, Department of Defense (Health Affairs), and Department of Veterans Affairs.

most benefit, should be linked with these databases. Such systems should provide relevant information about the patient and his or her medications to anyone who needs them. Bates et al.[62] report on the ability of computerized information systems to identify and prevent adverse events using three hierarchical levels of clinical information. Using only what they call Level 1 information (demographic information, results of diagnostic tests, and current medications), 53 percent of adverse events were judged identifiable. Using Level 2 (as well as Level 1) information (physician order entry), 58 percent were judged identifiable. Using Level 3 (as well as Levels 1 and 2) information that included additional clinical data such as automated problem lists, the authors judged that 89 percent of adverse events were identifiable. In this study a small but significant number of adverse events (5, 13, and 23 percent, respectively) were judged preventable by using such techniques as guided-dose, drug–laboratory, and drug–patient characteristic software algorithms.

As with any new technology, implementing any of these practices requires attention to the user–system interface to minimize the introduction of new problems. It is helpful if these systems have a clearly designated "process manager." It is also important to remember that on-line computer entry does not eliminate all errors associated with prescribing drugs. For example, if allergic reactions to a medication are not entered in the database for a given patient, the order entry system cannot alert the prescriber when the same medication (or one in the same class) is prescribed. Other errors such as transcription errors can remain if they are within an expected range.

Use Pharmaceutical Software

Pharmacies in health care organizations should routinely use reliable computer software programs designed to check all prescriptions for duplicate drug therapies; potential drug–drug and drug–allergy interactions; and out-of-range doses, timing, and routes of administration.

Software is available that permits pharmacists to check each new prescription at a minimum for dose, interactions with other medications the patient is taking, and allergies. Although not as sophisticated as computerized physician order entry, until the latter is in place, pharmacy computerized checking can be an efficient way to intercept prescribing errors. The committee cautions, however, that many pharmacy computer systems today are of limited reliability when used to detect and correct prescription errors, most notably serious drug interactions.[63] At a minimum, such systems should screen for duplicate prescriptions, patient allergies, potential drug–

drug interactions, out-of-range doses for patient weight or age, and drug–lab interactions. Because such pharmacy software may not be programmed to detect all, or even most, dangers, pharmacists and other personnel should not rely on these systems exclusively nor, on the other hand, habitually override alerts.

Implement Unit Dosing

If medications are not packaged in single doses by the manufacturer, they should be prepared in unit doses by the central pharmacy. Unit dosing—the preparation of each dose of each medication by the pharmacy—reduces handling as well as the chance of calculation and mixing errors. Unit dosing can reduce errors by eliminating the need for calculation, measurement, preparation, and handling on the nursing unit and by providing a fully labeled package that stays with the medication up to its point of use.

Unit dosing was a major systems change that significantly reduced dosing errors when it was introduced nearly 20 years ago. Unit dosing has been recommended by the American Society of Health-System Pharmacists, JCAHO, NPSF, and the MHA in their "Best Practice Recommendations." As a cost-cutting measure, unfortunately some hospitals have recently returned to bulk dosing, which means that an increase in dosing errors is bound to occur.

Have the Central Pharmacy Supply High-Risk Intravenous Medications

Having the pharmacy place additives in IV solutions or purchasing them already mixed, rather than having nurses prepare IV solutions on patient care units, reduces the chance of calculation and mixing errors. For example, one study showed that the error rate in mixing of IV drugs is 20 percent by nurses; 9 percent by pharmacies, and 0.3 percent by manufacturers. This recommendation is supported by the American Society of Health-System Pharmacists, the Institute for Safe Medication Practices, and the experience reported by Bates et al.[64]

Use Special Procedures and Written Protocols for the Use of High-Risk Medications

A relatively small number of medications carry a risk of death or serious injury when given in excessive dose. However, these include several of the most powerful and useful medications in the therapeutic armamentarium. Examples are heparin, warfarin, insulin, lidocaine, magnesium, muscle relaxants, chemotherapeutic agents, and potassium chloride (see below), dextrose injections, narcotics, adrenergic agents, theophylline, and immunoglobin.[65,66] Both to alert personnel to be especially careful and to ensure that dosing is appropriate, special protocols and processes should be used for these "high-alert" drugs. Such protocols might include written and computerized guidelines, checklists, preprinted orders, double-checks, special packaging, and labeling.

Do Not Store Concentrated Potassium Chloride Solutions on Patient Care Units

Concentrated potassium chloride (KCl) is the most potentially lethal chemical used in medicine. It is widely used as an additive to intravenous solutions to replace potassium loss in critically ill patients. Each year, fatal accidents occur when concentrated KCl is injected because it is confused with another medication. Because KCl is never intentionally used undiluted, there is no need to have the concentrated form stocked on the patient care unit. Appropriately diluted solutions of KCl can be prepared by the pharmacy and stored on the unit for use.

After enacting its sentinel event reporting system, JCAHO found that eight of ten incidents of patient death resulting from administration of KCl were the result of the infusion of KCl that was available as a floor stock item.[67] This has also been reported as a frequent cause of adverse events by the U.S. Pharmacopoeia (USP) Medication Errors Reporting Program.[68]

Ensure the Availability of Pharmaceutical Decision Support

Because of the immense variety and complexity of medications now available, it is impossible for nurses or doctors to keep up with all of the information required for safe medication use. The pharmacist has become an essential resource in modern hospital practice. Thus, access to his or her expertise must be possible at all times.[69,70] Health care organizations would greatly benefit from pharmaceutical decision support. When possible, medications should be dispensed by pharmacists or with the assistance of pharmacists. In addition, a substantial number of errors are made when nurses or other nonpharmacist personnel enter pharmacies during off hours to obtain drugs. Although small hospitals cannot afford and do not need to have a pharmacist physically present at all times, all hospitals must have access to pharmaceutical decision support, and systems for dispensing medications should be designed and approved by pharmacists.

Include a Pharmacist During Rounds of Patient Care Units

As the major resource for drug information, pharmacists are much more valuable to the patient care team if they are physically present at the time decisions are being made and orders are being written. For example, in teaching hospitals, medical staff may conduct "rounds" with residents and other staff. Pharmacists should actively participate in this process and be present on the patient care unit when appropriate. Such participation is usually well received by nurses and doctors, and it has been shown to significantly reduce serious medication errors. Leape et al.[71] measured the effect of pharmacist participation on medical rounds in the intensive care unit. They found that in one large, urban, teaching hospital the rate of preventable adverse drug events related to prescribing decreased significantly—66 percent—from 10.4 per 1,000 patient-days before the intervention to 3.5 after the intervention; the rate in the control group was unchanged.

Make Relevant Patient Information Available at the Point of Patient Care

Many organizations have implemented ways to make information about patients available at the point of patient care as well as ways to ensure that patients are correctly identified and treated. With medication administration, some inexpensive but useful strategies include the use of colored wristbands (or their equivalent) as a way to alert medical staff of medication allergies. Colored wristbands or their functional equivalent can alert personnel who encounter a patient anywhere in a hospital to check for an allergy before administering a medication. Using computer-generated MARs, can minimize transcription errors and legibility problems as well as provide flow charts for patient care.

Improper doses, mix-ups of drugs or patients, and inaccurate records are common causes of medication errors in daily hospital practice. Bar coding (or an electronic equivalent) is an effective remedy.[72] It is a simple way to ensure that the identity and dose of the drug are as prescribed, that it is being given to the right patient, and that all of the steps in the dispensing and administration processes are checked for timeliness and accuracy. Bar coding can be used not only by drug manufacturers, but also by hospitals to ensure that patients and their records match. The Colmercy-O'Neil VA Medical Center in Topeka, Kansas, reports, for example, a 70 percent reduction in medication error rates between September, 1995 and April, 1998 by using a system that included bar coding of each does, use of a hand-held laser bar code scanner, and a radio computer link.[73]

Improve Patients' Knowledge About Their Treatment

A major unused resource in most hospitals, clinics, and practices is the patient. Not only do patients have a right to know the medications they are receiving, the reasons for them, their expected effects and possible complications, they also should know what the pills or injections look like and how often they are to receive them. Patients should be involved in reviewing and confirming allergy information in their records.

Practitioners and staff in health care organizations should take steps to ensure that, whenever possible, patients know which medications they are receiving, the appearance of these medications, and their possible side effects.[74] They should be encouraged to notify their doctors or staff of discrepancies in medication administration or the occurrence of side effects. If they are encouraged to take this responsibility, they can be a final "fail-safe" step.

At the time of hospital discharge, patients should also be given both verbal and written information about the safe and effective use of their medications in terms and in a language they can understand.

Patient partnering is not a substitute for nursing responsibility to give the proper medication properly or for physicians to inform their patients, but because no one is perfect, it provides an opportunity to intercept the rare but predictable error. In addition to patients' informing their health care practitioner about their current medications, allergies, and previous adverse drug experiences, the National Patient Safety Partnership has recommended that patients ask the following questions before accepting a newly prescribed medication:[75]

• Is this the drug my doctor (or other health care provider) ordered? What are the trade and generic names of the medication?
• What is the drug for? What is it supposed to do?
• How and when am I supposed to take it and for how long?
• What are the likely side effects? What do I do if they occur?

• Is this new medication safe to take with other over-the-counter or prescription medication or with dietary supplements that I am already taking? What food, drink, activities, dietary supplements, or other medication should be avoided while taking this medication?

SUMMARY

This chapter has proposed numerous actions based on both good evidence and principles of safe design that health care organizations could take now or as soon as possible to substantially improve patient safety. These principles include (1) providing leadership; (2) respecting human limits in process design; (3) promoting effective team functioning; (4) anticipating the unexpected; and (5) creating a learning environment.

The committee's recommendations call for health care organizations and health care professionals to make continually improved patient safety a specific, declared, and serious aim by establishing patient safety programs with defined executive responsibility. The committee also calls for the immediate creation of safety systems that incorporate principles such as (1) standardizing and simplifying equipment, supplies, and processes; (2) establishing team training programs; and (3) implementing nonpunitive systems for reporting and analyzing errors and accidents within organizations. Finally, drawing on these principles and on strong evidence, the committee calls on health care organizations to implement proven medication safety practices.

REFERENCES

1. Reason, James T. Forward to *Human Error in Medicine,* Marilyn Sue Bogner, ed. Hillsdale, NJ: Lawrence Erlbaum Associates, 1994, p. xiv. Though ecologically unsound, the analogy is apt.

2. Chassin, Mark R.; Galvin, Robert W., and the National Roundtable on Health Care Quality. The Urgent Need to Improve Health Care Quality. Institute of Medicine National Roundtable on Health Care Quality. *JAMA.* 280:1000–1005, 1998.

3. Cook, Richard I. Two Years Before the Mast: Learning How to Learn About Patient Safety. Invited presentation. "Enhancing Patient Safety and Reducing Errors in Health Care," Rancho Mirage, CA, November 8–10, 1998.

4. Senders, John. "Medical Devices, Medical Errors and Medical Accidents," in *Human Error in Medicine,* Marilyn Sue Bogner, ed. Hillsdale, NJ: Lawrence Erlbaum Associates, 1994.

5. Van Cott, Harold. "Human Errors: Their Causes and Reduction," in *Human Error in Medicine,* Marilyn Sue Bogner, ed., Hillsdale, NJ: Lawrence Erlbaum Associates, 1994.

6. Van Cott, 1994.

7. MacCormack, George. Zeroing in on Safety Excellence—It's Good Business. http://www.dupont.com/safety/esn97-1/zeroin.html 5/27/99.

8. DuPont Safety Resources. Safety Pays Big Dividends for Swiss Federal Railways. http://www.dupont.com/safety/ss/swissrail22.html 5/3/99.

9. From "Executive Safety News" DuPont Safety Resources. http://www.dupont.com/safety/esn98-3.html 5/3/99.

10. Alcoa. Alcoa Environment, Health and Safety Annual Report. 1997.

11. Sagan, Scott D. *The Limits of Safety. Organizations, Accidents, and Nuclear Weapons*. Princeton, N.J.: Princeton University Press, 1993.

12. Weick, Karl E. and Roberts, Karlene H. Collective Mind in Organizations: Heedful Interrelating on Flight Decks. *Administrative Science Quarterly*. 38:357–381, 1993.

13. Rasmussen, Jens. Skills, rules, Knowledge: Signals, Signs, and Symbols and Other Distinctions in Human Performance Models. *IEEE Transactions: Systems, Man & Cybernetics* (SMC-13): 257–267, 1983.

14. Reason, James. *Human Error*. New York: Cambridge University Press, 1990.

15. Moray, Nevill. "Error Reduction as a Systems Problem," in *Human Error in Medicine*, ed., Marilyn Sue Bogner, Hillsdale, NJ: Lawrence Erlbaum Associates, 1994.

16. Van Cott, 1994.

17. Norman, Donald A. *The Design of Everyday Things*. NY: Doubleday/Currency, 1988.

18. Gaba, David; Howard, Steven K., and Fish, Kevin J. *Crisis Management in Anesthesiology*. NY: Churchill-Livingstone, 1994.

19. Committee on Quality Assurance in Office-Based Surgery. A Report to New York State Public Health Council and New York State Department of Health, June, 1999.

20. Berwick, Donald M. "Taking Action to Improve Safety: How to Increase the Odds of Success," Keynote Address, Second Annenberg Conference, Rancho Mirage, CA, November 8, 1998.

21. Haberstroh, Charles H. "Organization, Design and Systems Analysis," in *Handbook of Organizations,* J.J. March, ed. Chicago: Rand McNally, 1965.

22. Leape, Lucian L.; Kabcenell, Andrea; Berwick, Donald M., et al. *Reducing Adverse Drug Events*. Boston: Institute for Healthcare Improvement, 1998.

23. Institute of Medicine. *Guidelines for Clinical Practice. From Development to Use.* Marilyn J. Field and Kathleen N. Lohr, eds. Washington, D.C.: National Academy Press, 1992.

24. Leape, et al., 1998.

25. Leape, et al., 1998.

26. Leape, et al., 1998.

27. Leape, et al., 1998.

28. Leape, et al., 1998.

29. Hwang, Mi Y. *JAMA* Patient Page. Take Your Medications as Prescribed. *JAMA*. 282:298, 1999.

30. Blumenthal, David. The Future of Quality Measurement and Management in a Transforming Health Care System. *JAMA*. 278:1622–1625, 1997.

31. Sheridan, Thomas B. and Thompson, James M. "People Versus Computers in Medicine," in *Human Error in Medicine,* Marilyn Sue Bogner, ed., Hillsdale, NJ: Lawrence Erlbaum Associates, 1994.

32. Hyman, William A. "Errors in the Use of Medical Equipment," in *Human Error in Medicine,* Marilyn Sue Bogner, ed., Hillsdale, NJ: Lawrence Erlbaum Associates, 1994.

33. Senders, John W. "Medical Devices, Medical Errors, and Medical Accidents," in *Human Error in Medicine,* Marilyn Sue Bogner, ed., Hillsdale, NJ: Lawrence Erlbaum Associates, 1994.

34. Cook, Richard I. Two Years Before the Mast: Learning How to Learn About Patient Safety. "Enhancing Patient Safety and Reducing Errors in Health Care," Rancho Mirage, CA, November 8–10, 1998.

35. Leape, et al., 1998.

36. Helmreich, Robert L.; Chidester, Thomas R.; Foushee, H. Clayton, et al. How Effective is Cockpit Resource Managmeent Training? *Flight Safety Digest.* May:1–17, 1990.

37. Chopra,V.; Gesink, Birthe J.; deJong, Jan, et al. Does Training on an Anaesthesia Simulator Lead to Improvement in Performance? *Br J Anaesthesia.* 293–297, 1994.

38. Denson, James S. and Abrahamson, Stephen. A Computer-Controlled Patient Simulator. *JAMA.* 208:504–508, 1969.

39. Howard, Steven K.; Gaba, David, D.; Fish, Kevin J., et al. Anesthesia Crisis Resource Management Training: Teaching Anesthesiologists to Handle Critical Incidents. *Aviation, Space, and Environmental Medicine.* 63:763–769, 1992.

40. Spence, Alastair. A. The Expanding Role of Simulators in Risk Management. *Br J Anaesthesia.* 78:633–634, 1997.

41. Inaccurate Reporting of Simulated Critical Anaesthetic Incidents. *Br J Anaesthesia.* 78:637–641, 1997.

42. Helmreich, Robert L. and Davies, Jan M. Anaesthetic Simulation and Lessons to be Learned from Aviation. [Editorial]. *Canadian Journal of Anaesthesia.* 44:907–912, 1997.

43. Institute of Medicine. *The Computer-Based Patient Record. An Essential Technology for Health Care. Revised Edition.* Washington, DC: National Academy Press, 1997.

44. Tuggy, Michael L. Virtual Reality Flexible Sigmoidoscopy Simulator Training: Impact on Resident Performance. *J Am Board Fam Pract.* 11:426–433, 1998.

45. Leape, Lucian, L.; Woods, David D.; Hatlie, Martin, J., et al. Promoting Patient Safety and Preventing Medical Error. *JAMA.* 280:1444–1447, 1998.

46. Leape, Lucian L. Error in Medicine. *JAMA* 272:1851–1857, 1994.

47. Kizer, Kenneth W. *VHA's Patient Safety Improvement Initiative,* presentation to the National Health Policy Forum, Washington, D.C., May 14, 1999.

48. Nolan, Thomas. Presentation, IHI Conference, Orlando, FL, December, 1998.

49. Zimmerman, Jack E.; Shortell, Stephen M., et al. Improving Intensive Care: Observations Based on Organizational Case Studies in Nine Intensive Care Units: A Prospective, Multicenter Study. *Crit Care Med.* 21:1443–1451, 1993.

50. Shortell, Stephen M.; Zimmerman, Jack E.; Gillies, Robin R., et al. Continuously Improving Patient Care: Practical Lessons and an Assessment Tool From the National ICU Study. *QRB Qual Rev Bull.* 18:150–155, 1992.

51. Manasse, Henri R. Jr. Toward Defining and Applying a Higher Standard of Quality for Medication Use in the United States. *Am J Health System Pharm.* 55:374–379, 1995.

52. Lesar, Timothy S.; Briceland, Laurie; and Stein, Daniel S. Factors Related to Errors in Medication Prescribing. *JAMA.* 277:312–317, 1997.

53. Avorn, Jerry. Putting Adverse Drug Events into Perspective. *JAMA.* 277:341–342, 1997.

54. Healthcare Leaders Urge Adoption of Methods to Reduce Adverse Drug Events. News Release. National Patient Safety Partnership, May 12, 1999.

55. Massachusetts Hospital Association (Massachusetts Coalition for the Prevention of Medical Errors). "MHA Best Practice Recommendations to Reduce Medication Errors," Kirle, Leslie E.; Conway, James; Peto, Randolph, et al. http://www.mhalink.org/mcpme/recommend.htm.

56. Leape, et al., 1998.

57. Consensus Statement. American Society of Health-system Pharmacists. Top-Priority Actions for Preventing Adverse Drug Events in Hospitals. Recommendations of an Expert Panel. *Am J Health System Pharm.* 53:747–751, 1996.

58. Bates, David W.; Leape, Lucian L.; Cullen, David J., et al. Effect of Computerized Physician Order Entry and a Team Intervention on Prevention of Serious Medical Error. *JAMA.* 280:1311–1316, 1998.

59. Bates, 1998.

60. Evans, R. Scott; Pestotnik, Stanley L.; Classen, David C., et al. A Computer-Assisted Management Program for Antibiotics and Other Anti-Infective Agents. *N Engl J Med.* 338(4):232–238, 1997. See also: Schiff, Gordon D.; and Rucker, T. Donald. Computerized Prescribing: Building the Electronic Infrastructure for Better Medication Usage. *JAMA.* 279:1024–1029, 1998.

61. Bates, David W.; Spell, Nathan, Cullen; David J., et al. The Costs of Adverse Drug Events in Hospitalized Patients. *JAMA.* 227:307–311, 1997.

62. Bates, David W.; O'Neil, Anne C.; Boyle, Deborah, et. al. Potential Identifiablity and Preventability of Adverse Events Using Information Systems. *J American Informatics Assoc.* 5:404–411, 1994.

63. Institute for Safe Medication Practices. Over-reliance on Pharmacy Computer Systems May Place Patients at Great Risk. http://www.ismp.org/ISMP/MSAarticles/Computer2.html 6/01/99.

64. Bates, David W.; Cullen, David J.; Laird, Nan, et al. Incidence of Adverse Drug Events and Potential Adverse Drug Events. *JAMA.* 274:29–34, 1995.

65. Leape, Lucian L.; Kabcenell, Andrea; Berwick, Donald M., et al. *Reducing Adverse Drug Events.* Boston: Institute for Healthcare Improvement, 1998.

66. Cohen, Michael; Anderson, Richard W.; Attilio, Robert M., et al. Preventing Medication Errors in Cancer Chemotherapy. *Am J Health System Pharm.* 53:737–746, 1996.

67. Sentinel Event Alert. The Joint Commission on Accreditation of Healthcare Organizations, Oakbrook Terrace, IL: JCAHO, 1998.

68. Cohen, Michael. Important Error Prevention Advisory. *Hosp Pharmacists.* 32:489–491, 1997.

69. ASHP Guidelines on Preventing Medication Errors in Hospitals. *Am J Hospital Pharmacists.* 50:305–314, 1993.

70. Crawford, Stephanie Y. Systems Factors in the Reporting of Serious Medication Errors. Presentation at Annenburg Conference, Rancho Mirage, CA, November 8, 1998.

71. Leape, Lucian L.; Cullen, David J.; Clapp, Margaret D., et al. Pharmacist Participation on Physician Rounds and Adverse Drug Events in the Intensive Care Unit. *JAMA..* 282(3):267–270, 1999.

72. Top Priority Actions for Preventing Adverse Drug Events in Hospitals. Recommendations of an Expert Panel. *Am J Health System Pharm.* 53:747–751, 1996.

73. Gebhart, Fred. VA Facility Slashes Drug Errors Via Bar-Coding. *Drug Topics.* 1:44, 1999.

74. Joint Commission on Accreditation of Healthcare Organizations. *1998 Hospital Accreditation Standards.* Oakbrook Terrace, IL: Joint Commission, 1998.

75. Healthcare Leaders Urge Adoption of Methods to Reduce Adverse Drug Events. News Release. National Patient Safety Partnership, May 12, 1999.

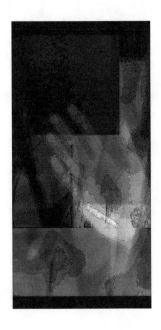

Appendixes

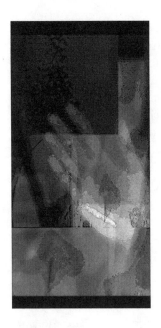

A
Background and
Methodology

This report on patient safety is part of a larger study examining the quality of health care in America. The Quality of Health Care in America project was initiated by the Institute of Medicine in June 1998, with the charge of developing a strategy that will result in a *threshold improvement* in quality over the next ten years. Specifically, the committee is charged with the following tasks:

- review and synthesis of findings in the literature pertaining to the quality of care provided in the health care system;
- development of a communications strategy for raising the awareness of the general public and key stakeholders of quality-of-care concerns and opportunities for improvement;
- articulation of a policy framework that will provide positive incentives to improve quality and foster accountability;
- identification of key characteristics and factors that enable or encourage providers, health care organizations, health plans, and communities to continuously improve the quality of care; and
- development of a research agenda in areas of continued uncertainty.

A growing body of rigorous research has documented serious and widespread quality problems in American medicine. The burden of harm conveyed by the collective impact of all of our health care quality problems requires the urgent attention of all stakeholders—the health professions, health policy makers, consumer advocates, and purchasers of care. The challenge is to bring the full potential benefit of effective health care to all Americans while avoiding unnecessary and harmful interventions and eliminating preventable complications of care. Meeting this challenge demands a readiness to think in radically new ways about how to deliver health care services and how to assess and improve their quality. Yet neither business leaders, medical leaders, policy makers, nor the public has a clear picture about whether different forms of financing and delivery of care have affected the quality of care and how best to structure financing, oversight, and delivery of care to improve quality.

The methods used for this study included a review of available literature, a commissioned paper, public testimony, a telephone survey, and input from targeted groups on specific issues. A review of the literature relied on published articles focusing on areas of quality, medical errors, patient safety, aviation safety, worker safety, and pharmaceutical safety. Working papers and web sites were also consulted, generally provided by organizations involved in patient safety, accreditation, and existing error reporting systems.

A paper was commissioned on the legal issues raised in protecting data and reporters in error reporting systems that are external to a health care organization. This paper was completed for the committee by Randall Bovbjerg, J.D., and David Shapiro, M.D., J.D. It formed the basis for Chapter 6 of this report.

The content of this report was discussed at seven meetings of two different subcommittees. It was on the agenda at four meetings of the Subcommittee on Creating an External Environment for Quality and three meetings of the Subcommittee on Creating the 21st Century Health System. It was also on the agenda at three meetings of the Committee on Quality of Health Care in America. The public testimony provided follows:

Subcommittee on Creating an External Environment for Quality

November 2, 1998   Martin Hatlie, National Patient Safety
                      Foundation
                      Michael Cohen, Institute for Safe Medication
                      Practices
                      Ronald Goldman, Veterans Health
                      Administration

January 29, 1999   Charles Billings, M.D., Ohio State University
                      (designer of the Aviation Safety Reporting
                      System)
June 15, 1999   Tim Cuerdon, Health Care Financing
                      Administration
                      Margaret VanAmringe, Joint Commission on
                      Accreditation of Health Care Organizations
                      Marge Keyes, Agency for Healthcare Research
                      and Quality

Joint Meeting of Both Subcommittees

June 16, 1999   Kenneth Kizer, M.D., Undersecretary of
                      Health, Veterans Health Administration

A short telephone survey was conducted between February 24 and May 5, 1999 of a number of states having error reporting systems that affect hospitals. The list of states was obtained from the Joint Commission on Accreditation of Healthcare Organizations. A nonrepresentative sample was chosen to obtain additional information on their programs, focusing mainly on the largest states. The respondent was the individual at the state health department with administrative responsibility over the reporting program. Information was collected on the definition of a reportable event, which organizations submit reports, the number of reports submitted in the most recent year available, the year the reporting program was implemented, who has access to the information reported, and what is done with the information obtained (e.g., organization follow-up on specific events, compilation of data and trending over time). All respondents were given an opportunity to review the information on their states and make any corrections or clarifications.

Finally, input was obtained through two group meetings with specific key audiences. The first meeting was a 90-minute discussion held on August 2, 1999, at the 12th Annual Conference of the National Academy for State Health Policy in Cincinnati, Ohio. This meeting was attended by 19 people, all of whom had responsibilities associated with quality-of-care issues, some related to state error reporting programs. Open discussion was held on roles that states can play in ensuring adequate oversight of quality-of-care and patient safety, and what would be helpful to the states to increase their efforts in safety oversight.

The second meeting was a one-day roundtable discussion held on September 9, 1999, with health professionals active in their professional societies and associations through support from The Commonwealth Fund. This meeting was attended by 14 people representing medicine, nursing, and pharmacy. This open discussion covered issues related to the extent to which the health and medical community is aware of quality and safety concerns, specific actions that professional societies and groups can take to improve patient safety, and barriers that impede these actions from moving forward.

OTHER IOM WORK ON QUALITY

This quality initiative represents a continuing IOM interest in quality of health care. Several other quality-of-care projects have been undertaken in recent years.

America's Health in Transition: Protecting and Improving the Quality of Health and Health Care (IOM-wide special initiative)

The Special Initiative on Health Care Quality was created in 1996 to examine how to maintain and improve the health and well-being of the population and the quality of care that the public receives as the health care system restructures. This special initiative is evaluating quality assessment and improvement tools and their uses, and promoting the application of appropriate tools at all levels of health care, in all organizations, for the entire population. The initiative will also inform consumers, policy makers, providers, and others of key opportunities and obstacles to achieving better health outcomes for individuals and populations, and will provide them with information and tools to enable them to make better decisions and choices about health and health care.

National Roundtable on Health Care Quality

The National Roundtable on Health Care Quality was created to examine continual changes in health care and the implications of these changes for the quality of health and health care in this nation. The Roundtable convened nationally prominent representatives of the private and public sectors (regional, state, and federal); academia; patients; and the health media to analyze unfolding issues concerning health care quality. This initiative produced three reports: *The Urgent Need to Improve Health Care Quality, Mea-*

suring the Quality of Health Care, and *Collaboration Among Competing Managed Care Organizations for Quality Improvement.*

Ensuring the Quality of Cancer Care

The National Cancer Policy Board undertook a comprehensive review of the quality of cancer care provided in the United States. The report, published in June 1999, delineates essential elements needed to improve quality in cancer care. The report provides an overview of the present cancer care system, moving from detection and early treatment to care at the end of life. Major obstacles impeding patient access to quality cancer care are identified. The report offers a model of an ideal cancer care delivery system and provides examples of the problems that limit early detection, accurate diagnosis, optimal treatment, and responsive supportive care. Recommendations to improve the quality of cancer care are offered for consideration by Congress, public and private health care purchasers, individual consumers, providers and researchers.

Improving Quality in Long-Term Care

The Committee on Improving Quality in Long-Term Care was convened to examine the means for assessing, overseeing, and improving the quality of long-term care in different settings and the practical and policy challenges of achieving a consistent quality of care regardless of where care is received. This study built on a 1986 report, *Improving the Quality of Care in Nursing Homes,* which initiated changes that significantly altered where long-term care is received and by whom. The most recent study examines the full range of long-term care settings and services, including nursing homes, assisted living facilities, and community-based home health care.

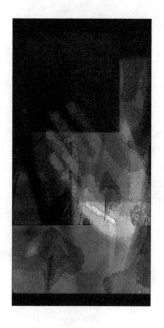

B
Glossary and Acronyms

GLOSSARY

Accident—An event that involves damage to a defined system that disrupts the ongoing or future output of the system.[1]

Active error—An error that occurs at the level of the frontline operator and whose effects are felt almost immediately.[2]

Adverse event—An injury resulting from a medical intervention.[3]

Bad outcome—Failure to achieve a desired outcome of care.

Error—Failure of a planned action to be completed as intended or use of a wrong plan to achieve an aim; the accumulation of errors results in accidents.

Health care organization—Entity that provides, coordinates, and/or insures health and medical services for people.

Human factors—Study of the interrelationships between humans, the tools they use, and the environment in which they live and work.[4]

Latent error—Errors in the design, organization, training, or maintenance that lead to operator errors and whose effects typically lie dormant in the system for lengthy periods of time.

Medical technology—Techniques, drugs, equipment, and procedures used by health care professionals in delivering medical care to individuals and the systems within which such care is delivered.[5]

Micro-system—Organizational unit built around the definition of repeatable core service competencies. Elements of a micro-system include (1) a core team of health care professionals, (2) a defined population of patients, (3) carefully designed work processes, and (4) an environment capable of linking information on all aspects of work and patient or population outcomes to support ongoing evaluation of performance.

Patient safety—Freedom from accidental injury; ensuring patient safety involves the establishment of operational systems and processes that minimize the likelihood of errors and maximizes the likelihood of intercepting them when they occur.

Quality of care—Degree to which health services for individuals and populations increase the likelihood of desired health outcomes and are consistent with current professional knowledge.[6]

Standard—A minimum level of acceptable performance or results *or* excellent levels of performance *or* the range of acceptable performance or results.[7] The American Society for Testing and Materials (ASTM) defines six types of standards:

1. Standard test methods—a procedure for identifying, measuring, and evaluating a material, product or system.
2. Standard specification—a statement of a set of requirements to be satisfied and the procedures for determining whether each of the requirements is satisfied.
3. Standard practice—a procedure for performing one or more specific operations or functions.
4. Standard terminology—a document comprising terms, definitions, descriptions, explanations, abbreviations, or acronyms.
5. Standard guide—a series of options or instructions that do not recommend a specific course of action.
6. Standard classification—a systematic arrangement or division of products, systems, or services into groups based on similar characteristics.[8]

System—Set of interdependent elements interacting to achieve a common aim. These elements may be both human and nonhuman (equipment, technologies, etc.).

ACRONYMS

ABMS	American Board of Medical Specialties
ADE	adverse drug event
AERS	Adverse Event Reporting System
AHRQ	Agency for Healthcare Research and Quality
AMA	American Medical Association
AMAP	American Medical Accreditation Program
ASHP	American Society of Health-System Pharmacists
ASRS	Aviation Safety Reporting System
ASTM	American Society for Testing and Materials
CABG	coronary artery bypass graft
CAHPS	Consumer Assessment of Health Plans
CDC	Centers for Disease Control
CEO	chief executive officer
CERT	Centers for Education and Research in Therapeutics
DRG	diagnosis-related group
FAA	Federal Aviation Administration
FDA	Food and Drug Administration
HCFA	Health Care Financing Administration
HEDIS	Health Plan Employer Data and Information Set
HIPAA	Health Insurance Portability and Accountability Act of 1996
HMO	health maintenance organization
HRSA	Health Resources and Services Administration
ICU	intensive care unit
ISMP	Institute for Safe Medication Practices
IV	intravenous
JCAHO	Joint Commission on Accreditation of Healthcare Organizations
MAR	Medical Administration Record
MER	Medical Error Reporting (system)
MERS-TM	Medical Event-Reporting System for Transfusion Medicine
M&M	morbidity and mortality
NASA	National Aeronautics and Space Administration

NCC-MERP	National Coordinating Council for Medication Error Reporting and Prevention
NCQA	National Committee for Quality Assurance
NIH	National Institutes of Health
NIOSH	National Institute for Occupational Safety and Health
NORA	National Occupational Research Agenda
NPSF	National Patient Safety Foundation
NTSB	National Transportation Safety Board
OPDRA	Office of Post-Marketing Drug Risk Assessment
OSHA	Occupational Safety and Health Administration
PICU	pediatric intensive care unit
POS	point of service
PPO	preferred provider organization
PRO	peer review organization
QIO	Quality Improvement Organization
QuIC	Quality Interagency Coordinating Committee
USP	U.S. Pharmacopeia
VHA	Veterans Health Administration

REFERENCES

1. Perrow, Charles. *Normal Accidents*. New York: Basic Books; 1984.

2. Reason, James T. *Human Error*. Cambridge, MA: Cambridge University Press; 1990.

3. Bates, David W.; Spell, Nathan; Cullen, David J., et al. The Costs of Adverse Drug Events in Hospitalized Patients. *JAMA*. 277:307–311, 1997.

4. Weinger, Matthew B.; Pantiskas, Carl; Wiklund, Michael, et al. Incorporating Human Factors into the Design of Medical Devices. *JAMA*. 280(17):1484, 1998.

5. Institute of Medicine. *Assessing Medical Technologies*. Washington, DC: National Academy Press; 1985.

6. Institute of Medicine. *Medicare: A Strategy for Quality Assurance*, Volume II. Washington, DC: National Academy Press; 1990.

7. Institute of Medicine, 1990.

8. American Society for Testing and Materials, www.astm.org/FAQ/3.html.

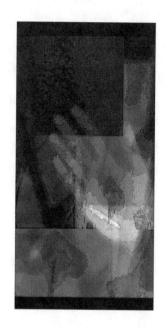

C
Literature Summary

This Appendix summarizes the literature described in Chapter 2. The references cited are at the end of Chapter 2.

TABLE C-1 Literature Summary

Reference	Sample Description	Data Source
General studies of errors and adverse events		
Thomas et al., forthcoming 2000	Randomly sampled 15,000 nonpsychiatric 1992 discharges from a representative sample of hospitals in Utah and Colorado.	Chart review by trained nurses and board-certified family practitioners and internists.
Bhasale et al., 1998 Analysing potential harm in Australian general practice	A non-random sample of 324 general practitioners reporting incidents between October 1993 and June 1995.	General practitioner-reported free-text descriptions of incidents and answered fixed-response questions.

Results	Definition(s)	Causes/Types of Error
Adverse events occurred in 2.9% ± 0.2 of hospitalizations in each state. 32.6% ± 4 of adverse events were due to negligence in Utah and 27.4 ± 2.4 were due to negligence in Colorado. Death occurred in 6.6% ± 1.2 of adverse events and 8.8% ± 2.5 of negligent adverse events. The leading cause of nonoperative adverse events were adverse drug events (19.3% of all adverse events; 35.1% were negligent). Operative events comprised 44.9% of all adverse events and 16.9% were negligent.	Adverse event—"an injury caused by medical management (rather than the disease process) that resulted in either a prolonged hospital stay or disability at discharge." Negligence was defined as "care that fell below the standard expected of physicians in their community."	46.1% of adverse events (22.3% negligent) were attributable to surgeons and 23.2% (44.9% negligent) were attributable to internists.
805 incidents were reported. 76% were preventable and 27% had potential for severe harm.	Incident—"an unintended event, no matter how seemingly trivial or commonplace, that could have harmed or did harm a patient."	Pharmacological management related to 51 per 100 incidents. Poor communication between patients and healthcare professionals and actions of others contributed to 23 per 100 incidents each. Errors in judgment contributed to 22 per 100 incidents.

Continued

TABLE C-1 *Continued*

Reference	Sample Description	Data Source

General studies of errors and adverse events *(continued)*

| Leape et al., 1993 Preventing medical injury | Record review of 1,133 patients who suffered from an adverse event (AE). | Harvard Medical Practice Study. |
| McGuire et al., 1992 Measuring and managing quality of surgery | 44,603 consecutive major operations performed at a large medical center from 1977 to 1990. | Resident reports giving name and procedure of each patient who suffered any complication. In a monthly conference, representatives of all specialties determined by consensus the category of each complication (inevitable, inherent risk, error, hospital deficit, coincidence, unknown). |

Results	Definition(s)	Causes/Types of Error
70% of adverse events were found to be preventable, 24% unpreventable, and 6% potentially preventable.	AE—per Leape (1991), AE is defined as "an unintended injury that was caused by medical management and that resulted in measurable disability." Preventable AE—an AE resulting from an error. Unpreventable AE—an AE resulting from a complication that cannot be prevented at the current state of knowledge. Potentially preventable AE—an AE where no error was identified but it is widely recognized that a high incidence of this type of complication reflects low standards of care or technical expertise.	The most common types of preventable errors were technical errors (44%), errors in diagnosis (17%), failures to prevent injury (12%), and errors in the use of a drug (10%). Approximately 20% of technical errors, 71% of diagnostic errors, 50% of preventative errors, and 37% of errors in the use of a drug were judged to be negligent.
2,428 patients (5.4%) suffered 2,797 complications (6.3%). 49% of these complications were attributable to error. 749 patients (1.7%) died during the same hospitalization. 7.5% of these deaths were attributable to error.		

Continued

TABLE C-1 *Continued*

Reference	Sample Description	Data Source

General studies of errors and adverse events *(continued)*

Reference	Sample Description	Data Source
Bedell et al., 1991 Incidence and characteristics of preventable iatrogenic cardiac arrests	203 patients who suffered from cardiac arrest at a teaching hospital during 1981.	At least one of the authors evaluated patients who underwent CPR within 24 hours of arrest. Information from the medical record was also used.
Leape et al., 1991 The nature of adverse events in hospitalized patients	30,195 randomly selected records in 51 hospitals in New York state (1984).	Hospital records.
DuBois et al., 1988 Preventable Deaths	182 deaths from 12 hospitals for 3 conditions (cerebrovascular accident, pneumonia, or myocardial infarction)	Investigators prepared a dictated summary of each patient's hospital course. Panels of 3 physicians for each condition then independently reviewed each summary and independently judged whether the death was preventable.

Results	Definition(s)	Causes/Types of Error
28 (14%) of arrests followed an iatrogenic complication. 17 (61%) of the 28 patients died. All 4 reviewers ● considered 18 (64%) of the iatrogenic arrests to have been preventable.	Iatrogenic cardiac arrest— "an arrest that resulted from a therapy or procedure or from a clearly identified error of omission."	The most common causes of potentially preventable arrest were medication errors and toxic effects (44%), and suboptimal response by physicians to clinical signs and symptoms (28%).
1,133 adverse events (AEs) occurred in 30,195 patients.	AE—"an unintended injury that was caused by medical management and that resulted in measurable disability."	Drug complications were the most common type of adverse event (19%), followed by wound infections (14%) and technical complications (13%). 58% of the adverse advents were errors in management, among which nearly half were attributable to negligence.
The physicians unanimously agreed that 14% of the deaths could have been prevented. 2 out of the 3 physicians found that 27% might have been prevented.		Preventable deaths from myocardial infarction reflected errors in management, from cerebrovascular accident reflected errors in diagnosis, and from pneumonia reflected errors in management and diagnosis.

Continued

TABLE C-1 *Continued*

Reference	Sample Description	Data Source

General studies of errors and adverse events *(continued)*

Steel et al., 1981 Iatrogenic illness on a general medical service at a university hospital	815 consecutive patients on a university hospital's general medical service during a 5-month period in 1979.	Record review, clinical personnel interviews, and information from utilization-review coordinators.
Cooper et al., 1978 Preventable anesthesia mishaps	47 interviews regarding preventable mishaps between September 1975 and April 1977 including staff and resident anesthesiologists from a large urban teaching hospital.	Interviewees selected at random from a list of departmental members.
Dripps et al., 1961 The role of anesthesia in surgical mortality	Records of 33,224 patients anesthetized in a 10-year period.	Patient records

Results	Definition(s)	Causes/Types of Error
36% of patients had an iatrogenic illness. 9% of the patients had an iatrogenic illness that threatened life or produced considerable disability while, in another 2%, the illness was believed to contribute to the death of the patient.	Iatrogenic illness—"any illness that resulted from a diagnostic procedure or from any form of therapy." In addition, the authors included harmful occurrences (e.g., injuries from a fall or decubitus ulcers) that were not natural consequences of the patient's disease.	
359 preventable critical incidents were identified and coded.	Critical incident—a mishap that "was clearly an occurrence that could have led (if not discovered or corrected in time) or did lead to an undesirable outcome, ranging from increased length of hospital stay to death or permanent disability."	82% of the preventable incidents reported involved human error and 14% involved equipment error.
12 of the 18,737 patients who received spinal anesthesia died from causes definitely related to the anesthetic (1:1,560). 27 of the 14,487 patients who received general anesthesia supplemented with a muscle relaxant died from causes directly related to the anesthetic (1:536).		

Continued

TABLE C-1 *Continued*

Reference	Sample Description	Data Source

General studies of errors and adverse events *(continued)*

Beecher and Todd, 1954 A study of the deaths associated with anesthesia and surgery based on a study of 599,548 anesthesias in ten institutions	All deaths from January 1, 1948, through December 31, 1952, occurring on the surgical services of 10 university hospitals.	1 team, consisting of an anesthesiologist, a surgeon, and a secretary, worked in each of the 10 hospitals and appraised the causes of all deaths on the surgical services.

Medication-related studies

Knox, 1999 Prescription errors tied to lack of advice *Globe* article	Analysis of medication errors by 51 Massachusetts pharmacists.	
Leape, 1999 Pharmacist participation on physician rounds and adverse drug events in the intensive care unit	75 patients randomly selected from each of 3 groups: all admissions to the study unit (2 medical ICUs at Massachusetts General Hospital) from February 1, 1993, through July 31, 1993 (baseline), and all admissions to the study unit (postintervention) and control unit from October 1, 1994, through July 7, 1995. 50 patients were also selected at random from the control unit during the baseline period.	Review of medical records and pharmacist recommendations.

Results	Definition(s)	Causes/Types of Error

7,977 of the 599,548 patients who received anesthesia died. Gross errors in anesthetic management occurred in 29 of the 384 (7.6%) deaths caused by anesthesia.

88% of medication errors involved the wrong drug or the wrong dose and 63% involved first-time prescriptions rather than refills.

Pharmacists cited factors that led to mistakes. 62% cited "too many telephone calls," 59% "unusually busy day," 53% "too many customers," 41% "lack of concentration," and 32% "staff shortage."

The rate of preventable adverse drug events (ADEs) due to ordering decreased by 66% from 10.4 per 1,000 patient days before the intervention to 3.5 per 1,000 patient days after the intervention. The rate was essentially unchanged during the same time periods in the control unit: 10.9 and 12.4 per 1,000 patient days.

ADE—per Bates (1993), ADE is defined as "an injury resulting from the administration of a drug."

Continued

TABLE C-1 *Continued*

Reference	Sample Description	Data Source
Medication-related studies *(continued)*		
Lazarou, 1998 Incidence of adverse drug reactions in hospitalized patients	39 prospective studies from U.S. hospitals.	4 electronic databases were searched for articles between 1966 and 1996.
Wilson et al., 1998 Medication errors in paediatric practice	682 children admitted to a Congenital Heart Disease Center at a teaching hospital in the United Kingdom.	Standardized incident report forms filled out by doctors, nurses, and pharmacists.
Andrews et al., 1997 An alternative strategy for studying adverse drug events	1,047 patients admitted to 3 units at a large, tertiary care, urban teaching hospital affiliated with a university medical school.	Ethnographers trained in qualitative observational research recorded all adverse events discussed while attending day-shift, weekday, regularly scheduled attending rounds, residents' work rounds, nursing shift changes, case conferences, and other scheduled meetings.

Results	Definition(s)	Causes/Types of Error
The overall incidence of serious adverse drug reactions (ADRs) in hospitalized patients was 6.7% and of fatal ADRs was 0.32%. In 1994, an estimated 2,216,000 hospitalized patients experienced serious ADRs and 106,000 had fatal ADRs, making these reactions the fourth and sixth leading causes of death.	ADR—"According to the World Health Organization definition, this is any noxious, unintended, and undesired effect of a drug, which occurs at doses in humans for prophylaxis, diagnosis, or therapy. This definition excludes therapeutic failures, intentional and accidental poisonings (i.e., overdose), and drug abuse. Also, this does not include adverse events due to errors in drug administration or noncompliance (taking more or less of a drug than the prescribed amount)."	
441 medical errors were reported. Prescription errors accounted for 68% of all reported errors, administration errors for 25%, and supply errors for 7%.	Medication error—"a mistake made at any stage in the provision of a pharmaceutical product to a patient."	Doctors accounted for 72% of the errors, nurses for 22%, pharmacy staff for 5%, and doctor/nurse combination for 1%
An adverse event occurred in 480 of the 1,047 patients (45.8%). 185 of the patients (17.7%) had at least one serious event. The likelihood of experiencing an adverse event increased approximately 6% for each day of a hospital stay. Only 1.2% of the patients experiencing serious events made claims to compensation.	Adverse event—a situation "in which an inappropriate decision was made when, at the time, an appropriate alternative could have been chosen."	Individuals caused 37.8% of adverse events while 15.6% of the events had interactive causes and 9.8% were due to administrative decisions.

Continued

TABLE C-1 *Continued*

Reference	Sample Description	Data Source

Medication-related studies *(continued)*

Reference	Sample Description	Data Source
Classen et al., 1997 Adverse drug events in hospitalized patients	Matched case-control study of all patients admitted to LDS Hospital (a tertiary care institution) from January 1, 1990, to December 31, 1993, and who had confirmed adverse drug events (ADEs). Controls and cases were matched on age, sex, acuity, year of admission, and primary discharge diagnosis related group (DRG).	Nursing acuity system and primary discharge DRG.
Cullen et al., 1997 Preventable adverse drug events in hospitalized patients	Prospective cohort study of 4,031 adult admissions to a stratified, random sample of 11 medical and surgical units (including 2 medical and 3 surgical ICUs and 4 medical and 2 surgical general care units) in 2 tertiary care hospitals over a 6-month period.	Stimulated self-report by nurses and pharmacists and daily review of all charts by nurse investigators. 2 independent reviewers classified the incidents.

Results	Definition(s)	Causes/Types of Error

ADEs complicated 2.43 per 100 admissions. The occurrence of an ADE was associated with an increased length of stay of 1.91 days and an increased cost of $2,262. The increased risk of death among patients experiencing an ADE was 1.88. Almost 50% of all ADEs are potentially preventable.

ADE—an event that is "noxious and unintended and occurs at doses used in humans for prophylaxis, diagnosis, therapy, or modification of physiologic functions."

The rate of preventable adverse drug events (ADEs) and potential ADEs in ICUs was 19 events per 1,000 patient days. This was nearly twice the rate of non-ICUs, but, when adjusted for the number of drugs used in the previous 24 hours or ordered since admission, there were no differences in rates between ICUs and non-ICUs.

ADE—"an injury resulting from medical intervention related to a drug." Potential adverse drug event— an incident "with potential for injury related to the use of a drug."

Continued

TABLE C-1 *Continued*

Reference	Sample Description	Data Source

Medication-related studies *(continued)*

Reference	Sample Description	Data Source
Lesar et al., 1997 Factors related to errors in medication prescribing	Every third prescribing error detected and averted by pharmacists in a 631-bed tertiary care teaching hospital between July 1, 1994, and June 30, 1995.	Retrospective evaluation by a physician and 2 pharmacists.
Schneitman-McIntire et al., 1996 Medication misadventures resulting in emergency department visits at an HMO medical center	Records of 62,216 patients who visited the emergency department of a California HMO between August 1992 and August 1993	Patient records and pharmacist interviews with patients.

Results	Definition(s)	Causes/Types of Error

2,103 errors thought to have potential clinical importance were detected, and the overall rate of errors was 3.99 errors per 1,000 medication orders.

The most common factors associated with errors were decline in renal or hepatic function requiring alteration of drug therapy (13.9%), patient history of allergy to the same medication class (12.1%), using the wrong drug name, dosage, form, or abbreviation (11.4% for both brand and generic name orders), incorrect dosage calculations (11.1%), and atypical or unusual and critical dosage frequency considerations (10.8%). The most common group factors associated with errors were those related to knowledge and the application of knowledge regarding drug therapy (30%); knowledge and use of knowledge regarding patient factors that affect drug therapy (29.2%); use of calculations, decimal points, or unit and rate expression factors (17.5%); and nomenclature factors, such as incorrect drug name, dosage form, or abbreviation (13.4%).

1,074 or 1.7% of the emergency department visits were due to medication misadventures. Of the 1,074 misadventures, 152 (14.1%) resulted in hospital admissions.

Misadventures "included noncompliance and inappropriate prescribing but excluded intentional overdoses and substance abuse."

Continued

TABLE C-1 *Continued*

Reference	Sample Description	Data Source

Medication-related studies *(continued)*

| Bates et al., *J Gen Intern Med*, 1995 Relationship between medication errors and adverse drug events | A cohort of 379 consecutive admissions during a 51-day period in three medical units of an urban tertiary care hospital. | Self-report by pharmacists, nurse review of all patient charts, and review of all medication sheets. 2 independent reviewers classified the incidents. |
| Bates et al., *JAMA*, 1995 Incidence of adverse drug events and potential adverse drug events | 4,031 adult admissions to a stratified random sample of 11 medical and surgical units in Brigham and Women's Hospital (726 beds) and Massachusetts General Hospital (846 beds) in Boston over a 6-month period between February and July 1993. | Stimulated self-reports by nurses and pharmacists and daily chart review. 2 independent reviewers classified the incidents. |

Results	Definition(s)	Causes/Types of Error
10,070 medication orders were written, and 530 medication errors were identified (5.3 errors/100 orders). 25 adverse drug events (ADEs) and 35 potential ADEs were found. 20% of the ADEs were associated with medication errors; all were judged preventable. 5 of 530 (0.9%) medication errors resulted in ADEs. Physician computer order entry could have prevented 86% of potential ADEs, 84% of non-missing dose medication errors, and 60% of preventable ADEs.	ADE—an injury "resulting from medical interventions related to a drug." Potential ADE—a medication error "with potential for injury but in which no injury occur-red." Medication error—an error "in the process of ordering or delivering a medication, regardless of whether an injury occurred or the potential for injury was present."	
247 adverse drug events (ADEs) and 194 potential ADEs were identified. Extrapolated event rates were 6.5 ADEs and 5.5 potential ADEs per 1,000 nonobstetrical admissions, for mean numbers per hospital per year of approximately 1,900 ADEs and 1,600 potential ADEs. 1% of all ADEs were fatal, 12% life-threatening, 30% serious, and 57% significant. 28% of all ADEs were judged preventable.	ADE—"an injury resulting from medical intervention related to a drug." Potential ADE—an incident "with potential for injury related to a drug."	56% of preventable ADEs occurred at the ordering stage, 34% at administration, 6% during transcription, and 4% during dispensing.

Continued

TABLE C-1 *Continued*

Reference	Sample Description	Data Source
Medication-related studies *(continued)*		
Cullen et al., 1995 The incident reporting system does not detect adverse drug events	All patients admitted to five patient care units in an academic tertiary care hospital between February and July 1993.	Consensus voting by senior hospital administrators, nursing leaders, and staff nurses.
Leape et al., 1995 Systems analysis of adverse drug events	All nonobstetric adult admissions to 11 medical and surgical units in 2 tertiary care hospitals in the period between February and July 1993.	Reports from each unit solicited daily by trained nurse investigators and peer interviews. 2 independent reviewers classified the incidents.
Willcox et al., 1994 Inappropriate drug prescribing for the community dwelling elderly	6,171 adults from a cross-sectional survey of a national probability sample of individuals aged 65 or older.	1987 National Medical Expenditure Survey.

Results	Definition(S)	Causes/Types of Error
Incident reports were submitted to the hospital's quality assurance program or called into the pharmacy hotline for 3 of the 54 people experiencing adverse drug events (ADEs). 15 (28%) of the ADEs were preventable and 26 (48%) were serious or life-threatening.	ADE—"an injury resulting from the use of a drug."	
334 errors were detected as the causes of 264 preventable adverse drug events (ADEs) and potential ADEs.	Potential ADEs—"errors that have the capacity to cause injury, but fail to do so, either by chance or because they are intercepted."	16 major system failures were identified as the causes of the errors, of which the most common was dissemination of drug knowledge (29% of 334 errors). 7 systems failures accounted for 78% of errors.
23.5% of people aged 65 years or older, or 6.64 million Americans, received at least 1 of the 20 contra-indicated drugs in 1987. 20.4% received two or more such drugs.	Contraindicated drugs include: 1) chlordiazepoxide 2) diazepam 3) flurazepam 4) meprobamate 5) pentobarbital 6) secobarbital 7) amitriptyline 8) indomethacin 9) phenylbutazone 10) chlorpropamide 11) propoxyphene 12) pentazocine 13) cyclandelate 14) isoxsuprine 15) dipyridamole 16) cyclobenzaprine 17) orphenidrat 18) methocarbamol 19) carisoprodol 20) trimethobenzamide	

Continued

TABLE C-1 *Continued*

Reference	Sample Description	Data Source
Medication-related studies *(continued)*		
Bates et al., 1993 Incidence and preventability of adverse drug events in hospitalized adults	All patients admitted to 2 medical, 2 surgical, and 2 obstetric general care units and 1 coronary intensive care unit over a 37-day period in an urban tertiary care hospital.	Records entered into logs in each unit and satellite pharmacies by nurses and pharmacists, reports solicited by a research nurse twice daily on each unit, and chart review by the nurse.
Einarson, 1993 Drug-related hospital admissions	English–language studies of humans admitted to the hospital because of adverse drug reactions (ADRs) resulting from a patient's noncompliance or unintentionally inappropriate drug use.	Manual and computerized literature searches using MEDLINE, *Index Medicus*, and *International Pharmaceutical Abstracts* as databases

Results	Definition(s)	Causes/Types of Error
73 drug-related incidents occurred in 2,967 patient days. 27 incidents were judged adverse drug events (ADEs), 34 potential ADEs, and 12 problem orders. 5 of the 27 ADEs were life-threatening, 9 were serious, and 13 were significant. 15 of the 27 ADEs (57%) were judged definitely or probably preventable.	ADE—"an injury resulting from the administration of a drug." Potential ADE—an incident "with a potential for injury related to a drug . . . [and an incident] in which a potentially harmful order was written but intercepted before the patient actually received the drug." Problem order—"an incident in which a drug-related error was made, but was judged not to have the potential for injury."	Physicians caused 72% of the incidents, with the remainder divided evenly between nursing, pharmacy, and clerical personnel.
Between 1996 and 1989, adverse drug reaction (ADR) rates from 49 hospitals or groups of hospitals in international settings were published in 37 articles. Drug-induced hospitalizations account for approximately 5% of all admissions. Reported admissions caused by ADRs ranged from 0.2% to 21.7%, with a median of 4.9% and a mean of 5.5%. 3.7% of patients admitted for ADRs died.	ADR—"any unintended or undesired consequence of drug therapy." Noncompliance—"any deviation from the regimen written (and intended) by the prescriber."	11 reports indicated that noncompliance induced 22.7% of ADR hospitalizations.

Continued

TABLE C-1 *Continued*

Reference	Sample Description	Data Source

Medication-related studies *(continued)*

Brennan et al., 1991 Incidence of adverse events and negligence in hospitalized patients	30,195 randomly selected records in 51 hospitals in New York state (1984).	Hospital records.
Classen et al., 1991 Computerized surveillance of adverse drug events in hospital patients	36,653 hospitalized patients in the LDS Hospital, Salt Lake City between May 1, 1989, and October 31, 1990.	Integrated hospital information system and pharmacist review of medical records.
Beers et al., 1990 Potential adverse drug interactions in the emergency room	424 randomly selected adults who visited the emergency room at a university-affiliated hospital. All subjects were discharged without hospital admission.	Complete emergency department record on every patient.

Results	Definition(s)	Causes/Types of Error

Adverse events (AEs) occurred in 3.7% of the hospitalizations. Although 70.5% gave rise to disabilities lasting less than 6 months, 2.6% of the adverse events caused permanently disabling injuries and 13.6% resulted in death.

AE—"an injury that was caused by medical mismanagement (rather than the underlying disease) and that prolonged the hospitalization, produced a disability at the time of discharge, or both."

731 verified adverse drug events (ADEs) occurred in 648 patients. 701 ADEs were classified as moderate or severe. Physicians, pharmacists, and nurses voluntarily reported 92 of the 731 ADEs detected using the automated system. The remaining 631 were detected from automated signals, the most common of which were diphenhydramine hydrochloride and naloxone hydrochloride use, high serum drug levels, leukopenia, and the use of phytonadione and antidiarrheals.

ADE—an event that is "noxious and unintended and occurs at doses used in man for prophylaxis, diagnosis, therapy, or modification of physiologic functions." "Therapeutic failures, poisonings, and intentional overdoses" were excluded.

47% of visits led to added medication. In 10% of the visits in which at least one medication was added, a new medication added a potential adverse interaction.

"Drug interactions are an aspect of the inappropriate use of medication that may endanger patients and that may be avoided by more careful prescribing."

Continued

TABLE C-1 *Continued*

Reference	Sample Description	Data Source
Medication-related studies *(continued)*		
Hallas et al., 1990 Drug related admissions to a cardiology department	366 consecutive patients admitted to the cardiology department at Odense University Hospital, Denmark, during a 2-month period (May–June 1988).	Written and verbal histories and blood samples.
Lesar et al., 1990 Medication prescribing errors in a teaching hospital	289,411 medication orders written between January 1, 1987, and December 31, 1987, in a tertiary care teaching hospital.	Medication orders reviewed by a centralized staff of pharmacists and the prescribing physicians.
Sullivan et al., 1990 Noncompliance with medication regimens and subsequent hospitalizations	7 studies and 2,942 admissions with comparable methodologies and evaluation regarding the extent and direct cost of hospital admissions related to drug therapy noncompliance.	Meta-analytic literature review.

Results	Definition(s)	Causes/Types of Error
"Definite" or "probable" drug events accounted for 15 admissions, or a 4.1% drug-related hospitalization rate. 11 were due to adverse drug reactions (ADRs) and 4 to dose-related therapeutic failures (DTFs). Of these 15 admissions, 5 cases were judged to have been "definitely avoidable."	ADR—"any unintended and undesirable effect of a drug." DTF—"lack of therapeutic effect that could be linked causally to either too low a prescribed dose, noncompliance, recent dose reduction/discontinuation, interaction or inadequate monitoring."	Of the 15 admissions, 5 were considered to be due to a prescription error.
905 prescribing errors were detected and averted, of which 57.7% had a potential for adverse consequences. The overall error rate was 3.13 errors for each 1,000 orders written and the rate of significant errors was 1.81 per 1,000 orders.	Medication errors— "medication orders for the wrong drug, inappropriate dosage, inappropriate frequency, inappropriate dosage form, inappropriate route, inappropriate indication, ordering of unnecessary duplicate/ redundant therapy, contraindicated therapy, medications to which the patient was allergic, orders for the wrong patient, or orders missing information required for the dispensing and administration of the drug."	
5.5% of admissions can be attributed to drug therapy noncompliance, amounting to 1.94 million admissions. This represents $8.5 billion in unnecessary hospital expenditures in 1986, an estimated 1.7% of all health care expenditures that year.	Drug therapy noncompliance— includes overuse, underuse, and erratic use of drugs.	

Continued

TABLE C-1 *Continued*

Reference	Sample Description	Data Source

Medication-related studies *(continued)*

| Raju et al., 1989 Medication errors in neonatal and paediatric intensive-care units | 2,147 patients admitted to a 17-bed NICU and 7-bed PICU (1,224 to NICU [57%] and 923 to PICU [43%]) at the University of Illinois Hospital from January 1985 to December 1988. | Written incident reports submitted by the individual who noticed the error. |
| Blum et al., 1988 Medication error prevention by pharmacists | Orders written between November 1986 and February 1987 at Indiana University Hospitals that contained potential medication errors about which the physician had been contacted. | Carbon copies of orders saved by pharmacists in the pediatric and adult facilities and reviewed by the four co-authors that served as the study monitors. |

Results	Definition(s)	Causes/Types of Error
315 iatrogenic medication errors were reported among the 2,147 neonatal and pediatric care admissions, an error rate of 1 per 6.8 admissions (14.7%). The frequency of iatrogenic injury of any sort due to a medication error was 3.1%, or 1 for each 33 intensive care admissions. 66 errors resulted in injury, 33 were potentially serious, 32 caused mild injuries, and 1 patient suffered acute aminophylline poisoning.	Medication error—"a dose of medication that deviates from the physicians' order as written in the medical record. . . . Except for error of omission, the medication dose must actually reach the patient . . . a wrong dose (or other type of error) that is detected and corrected before administration will not constitute a medication error. . . . Prescription errors (not dispensed and administered to the patient) . . . are excluded from this definition . . ."	60.3% of the 315 errors were attributable to nurses and 29.6% to pharmacists. Only 2.9% were attributable to physicians (because prescription errors detected before drug administration were not counted).
123,367 medication orders were written. Riley Hospital for Children had 1,277 errors out of the 48,034 (2.7%) orders written and University Hospital had 1,012 errors out of 75,333 (1.3%) orders written. 90.4% of the overall orders questioned by pharmacists were confirmed by the physician as being in error. 0.2% of the 2289 errors were classified as potentially lethal, 13.7% were serious, 34.2% were significant, and 51.9% were minor. The number of errors that pharmacists prevent each year approaches 9,000.	Order with a potential medication error—"if any aspect of the order was not in accordance with information in standard reference text, an approved protocol, or dosing guidelines approved by the pharmacy and therapeutics committee of the hospitals."	

Continued

TABLE C-1 *Continued*

Reference	Sample Description	Data Source

Medication-related studies *(continued)*

Nolan and O'Malley, 1988 Prescribing for the elderly, part I	21 hospital inpatient studies conducted in the United States, United Kingdom, Israel, New Zealand, Switzerland, Canada, and India published between 1964 and 1981.	Review of published studies on adverse drug reactions (ADRs).
Folli et al., 1987 Medication error prevention by clinical pharmacists in two children's hospitals	101,022 medication orders prescribed in two children's teaching hospitals (Miller Children's Hospital of Memorial Medical Center [MMC] and Stanford University Medical Center [SUMC]) during a six-month period (February through July 1985).	Copies of errant chart orders reviewed by a member of the pediatric faculty or attending physician and by two pediatric clinical pharmacist practitioners.
Perlstein et al., 1979 Errors in drug computations during newborn intensive care	43 nursing, pharmacy, and medical personnel tested for accuracy in calculating drug doses to be administered to newborn infants. (27 registered nurses, 5 registered pharmacists, and 11 pediatricians.)	

Results	Definition(s)	Causes/Types of Error

Rates of patients experiencing ADRs ranged from 1.5% to 43.5%. A majority of the studies documented ADR rates between 10% and 25%.

A combined total of 479 errant medication orders were identified at the two institutions. MMC and SUMC had similar frequency of error, 4.9 and 4.5 errors per 1,000 medication orders, or 1.37 and 1.79 per 100-patient days, respectively. Involving pharmacists in the reviewing of drug orders reduced the potential harm resulting from errant medication orders significantly.

Errant medication order— "An order was considered to be potentially in error if it was not in accordance with standard pediatric references, current published literature, or dosing guidelines approved by the pharmacy and therapeutics committees of each hospital."

The most common type of error was incorrect dosage. The most prevalent type of error was overdosage.

The mean test score for nurses was 75.6%. 56% of the errors would have resulted in administered doses ten times greater or less than the ordered dose. The mean test score was 96% for pharmacists and none of the errors would have resulted in the administration of doses over 1% greater or less than the dose ordered. Pediatricians averaged a score of 89.1%. 38.5% of the errors would have resulted in the administration of doses ten times higher or lower than the dose ordered.

Continued

TABLE C-1 *Continued*

Reference	Sample Description	Data Source

Medication-related studies *(continued)*

Miller, 1977
Interpretation of studies on
adverse drug reactions

Boston Collaborative Drug
Surveillance Program

Burnum, 1976
Preventability of adverse
drug reactions

1,000 adult medical patients
drawn from a community,
office-based practice of
general internal medicine.

Physician observation.

Jick, 1974
Drugs: remarkably
nontoxic

19,000 inpatients admitted
to medical wards.

Boston Collaborative Drug
Surveillance Program

Results	Definition(s)	Causes/Types of Error

Adverse drug reactions (ADRs) occur in approximately 30% of hospitalized patients and after about 5% of drug exposures. The rate per patient of life-threatening ADRs in 3% and the rate per course of drug therapy is 0.4%.

Adverse drug reactions (ADRs) occurred in 42 of the individual patients. 23 (55%) were judged unnecessary and potentially preventable.

23% of the 42 ADRs were attributable to physician error (10 out of 42; 6 because of giving a drug that was not indicated and 4 because of improper drug administration), 17% to patient or pharmacist error, and 14% to errors shared by the physician, patient and pharmacist.

30% of hospitalized medical patients have at least 1 adverse drug reaction (ADR) while hospitalized. An estimated 3 million hospital patients have an ADR in medical units each year.

Continued

TABLE C-1 *Continued*

Reference	Sample Description	Data Source
Medication-related studies *(continued)*		
Phillips et al., 1974 Increase in U.S. Medication-error deaths between 1983 and 1993		All United States death certificates between 1983 and 1993.
Talley and Laventurier, 1974 Drug-induced illness		Boston Collaborative Drug Surveillance Program and an Israeli study.
Cost		
Thomas et al., 1999	Medical records of 14,732 randomly selected 1992 discharges from 28 hospitals in Utah and Colorado	Two-stage chart review by trained nurses and board-certified family practitioners and internists.

Results	Definition(s)	Causes/Types of Error

In 1983, 2,876 people died from medication errors. By 1993, this number had risen to 7,391, a 2.57-fold increase. Between 1983 and 1993, outpatient medication error deaths rose 8.48-fold (from 172 to 1,459) and inpatient medical error deaths rose 2.37-fold (504 to 1,195).

Medication errors—"'accidental poisoning by drugs, medicaments, and biologicals' and have resulted from acknowledged errors, by patients or medical personnel."

An estimated incidence of lethal adverse drug reactions ranges from a low of 60,000 (.18% incidence) to a high of 140,000 (.44% incidence) for hospitalized patients in the U.S.

459 adverse events were detected, of which 265 were preventable. Death occurred in 6.6% of adverse events and 6.9% of preventable adverse events. The total costs were $661,889,000 for adverse events and $308,382,000 for preventable adverse events. Health care costs were $348,081,000 for all adverse events and $159,245,000 for preventable adverse events. 57% of the adverse event health care costs and 46% of the preventable adverse event costs were attributable to outpatient medical care.

Adverse event—"an injury caused by medical management (rather than the disease process) that resulted in either prolonged hospital stay or disability at time of discharge."

Continued

TABLE C-1 *Continued*

Reference	Sample Description	Data Source
Cost (continued)		
Bates et al., 1997 The costs of adverse drug events in hospitalized patients	4,108 admissions to a stratified random sample of 11 medical and surgical units in Brigham and Women's Hospital (726 beds) and Massachusetts General Hospital (846 beds) in Boston over a 6-month period between February and July 1993. Cases were patients with an adverse drug event (ADE), and the control for each case was a patient on the same unit as the case with the most similar pre-event length of stay.	Stimulated self-reports by nurses and pharmacists and daily chart review. 2 independent reviewers classified the incidents.
Bootman et al., 1997 The health care cost of drug-related morbidity and mortality in nursing facilities	To estimate the cost of drug-related problems (DRPs) within nursing facilities, a decision analysis technique was used to develop a probability pathway model.	Survey of an expert panel consisting of consultant pharmacists and physicians with practice experience in nursing facilities and geriatric care.

Results	Definition(s)	Causes/Types of Error
247 ADEs occurred among 207 admissions and 60 were preventable. The additional length of stay was 2.2 days with an ADE and 4.6 days with a preventable ADE. The estimated post-event costs attributable to an ADE were $2,595 for all ADEs and $4,685 for preventable ADEs. The estimated annual costs for a 700-bed teaching hospital attributable to all ADEs are $5.6 million and to preventable ADEs are $2.8 million. The national hospital costs of ADEs was estimated at $4 billion; preventable ADEs alone would cost $2 billion.	ADE—"an injury resulting from medical intervention related to a drug." Potential ADE—"incidents in which an error was made but no harm occurred."	
The cost of drug-related morbidity and mortality with the services of consultant pharmacists was $4 billion compared with $7.6 billion without services of consultant pharmacists. For every dollar spent on drugs in nursing facilities, $1.33 is consumed in the treatment of DRPs.	DRPs—"an event of circumstance involving a patient's drug treatment that actually or potentially interferes with the achievement of an optimal outcome."	

Continued

TABLE C-1 *Continued*

Reference	Sample Description	Data Source

Cost (continued)

Johnson and Bootman, 1995 Drug-related morbidity and mortality	A probability pathway model was developed for drug-related morbidity and mortality based primarily on drug-related problems (DRPs). A panel of experts gave estimates on the numbers of patients affected by DRPs and monetary value data were taken from published reports and statistical reports.	Telephone survey of 15 expert practicing pharmacists.
Schneider et al., 1995 Cost of medication-related problems at a university hospital	109 patients at a university-affiliated medical center hospital who were known to have had clinical consequences from an adverse drug reaction (ADR) or medication error.	Retrospective chart review.
Bloom, 1988 Cost of treating arthritis and NSAID-related gastrointestinal side-effects	Retrospective analysis of all direct costs related to the care of 527 Medicaid recipients treated for arthritis with non-steroidal anti-inflammatory drugs (NSAIDs) between December 1, 1981 and November 30, 1983.	Medicaid Management Information System of Washington, D.C.

Results	Definition(s)	Causes/Types of Error
Drug-related morbidity and mortality costs an estimated $76.6 billion in the ambulatory setting in the United States. The panel members estimated that 40% of patients who receive drug therapy would have some form of DRP.	Drug-related problem— "an event or circumstance that involves a patient's drug treatment that actually, or potentially, interferes with the achievement of an optimal outcome."	
349 clinical outcomes associated with medical related problems (MRPs) (average of approximately 3 outcomes per patient) were detected. For the 1,911 ADRs and medication errors reported through the voluntary reporting system in 1994, the estimated annual cost was just under $1.5 million.		
In 1983, an estimated $3.9 million was spent on treating preventable gastrointestinal adverse drug reactions to NSAIDs.	Gastrointestinal adverse drug reaction—"any claim for payment accompanied by a diagnosis of peptic ulcer, gastritis/duodenitis, other disorders of the stomach or duodenum, gastrointestinal symptoms, or a pharmacy claim for an H2-recepter antagonist, sucralfate or antacid, which occurred during the arthritis treatment study period.	

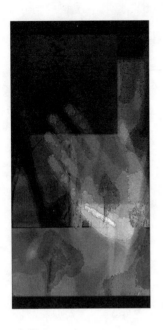

D
Characteristics of State Adverse Event Reporting Systems

CALIFORNIA

Reportable event   Occurrences such as epidemic outbreaks, poisonings, fires, major accidents, death from unnatural causes, or other catastrophes and unusual occurrences that threaten the welfare, safety, or health of patients, personnel, or visitors. Other occurrences include, but are not limited to, prevalence of communicable disease; infestation by parasites or vectors; disappearance or loss of a patient or inmate-patient; sexual acts involving patients who are minors; nonconsenting adults, or persons incapable of consent; physical assaults on inmate-patients, employees, or visitors; and all suspected criminal activity involving inmate-patients, employees, or visitors.

Who submits reports   General acute care hospitals, acute psychiatric hospitals, skilled nursing facilities, immediate care facilities, home health agencies, primary care clinics, psychology clinics, psychiatric health facilities, adult day health centers, chemical dependency recovery hospitals, and correctional treatment centers.

Number of reports   4,337 (1998)

Year initiated   1972 (approximately)

Mandatory or voluntary   Mandatory; must be submitted within 24 hours of the incident.

Access to information   Reports that do not contain confidential information are accessible to the public. Reports that do contain confidential information can be obtained only by subpoena. The local licensing and certification office handles all requests for copies of reports.

Use of information   The state reviews the reported event and determines if an onsite visit is warranted. If violations of the regulations are suspected an onsite visit is conducted. If deficiencies are noted the facility must submit an acceptable plan of correction. Violation of regulations can also result in state or federal citations. Civil penalties of up to $50 per day or enforcement actions can be imposed.

COLORADO

Reportable event   All deaths arising from unexplained causes or under suspicious circumstances. Brain and spinal cord injuries. Life-threatening complications of anesthesia. Life-threatening transfusion errors or reactions. Burns; missing persons; physical, sexual, and verbal abuse; neglect, misappropriation of property; diverted drugs; malfunction or misuse of equipment.

Who submits reports   All state-licensed health care facilities.

Number of reports   1,233 (1998)

Year initiated   1989

Mandatory or voluntary   Mandatory under Colorado State Statute 25-1-124(2).

Access to information   The name of the facility is disclosed. Patient and personnel information is kept confidential. Report summaries are posted on the Internet once the facility investigation is complete.

Use of information   An advisory committee meets monthly to identify patterns and issues. Summaries of the reviewed reports are sent out to the facilities and they have seven days to comment. The state will issue deficiencies if deemed necessary. All information is entered into a computer program for tracking. Surveyors and investigators review the information in the institution-specific database prior to conducting the regular survey and complaint investigations.

CONNECTICUT

Reportable event   All accidents or incidents that resulted in serious injury, death, or disruption of facility services.

Who submits reports   Nursing homes and hospitals.

Number of reports   14,783 (1996)—approximately 14,000 from nursing homes.

Year initiated   1987

Mandatory or voluntary   Mandatory for nursing homes; voluntary for hospitals.

Access to information   Reports disclose the name of the facility, but no information on patients or personnel. To obtain a report, one must fill out a Freedom of Information Act form and submit the request to the health department.

Use of information   Information is reviewed by a nurse consultant who determines if there needs to be an investigation by the health department.

FLORIDA

Reportable event	Urgent issue: life-threatening situation, epidemic outbreak. Code 15: serious adverse event (i.e., wrongful death, brain injury, wrong limb removal, incorrect surgery).
Who submits reports	Hospitals and ambulatory surgical centers.
Number of reports	Approximately 5,000 a year; 4,000 are urgent issue and 1,000 are Code 15.
Year initiated	1985
Mandatory or voluntary	Mandatory
Access to information	A summary of the aggregate data collected from reports is issued once a year. All other information is confidential and cannot be released without a subpoena.
Use of information	Urgent-issue situations are considered to be outside the facility's control; and thus no facility follow-up is required. When reporting a Code 15, an analysis of the injury and a plan of correction must be submitted by the facility within 15 days. The state's risk management program tracks trends in the reporting.

KANSAS

Reportable event	An act by a health care provider that (1) is or may be below the applicable standard of care and has a reasonable probability of causing injury to a patient or (2) may be grounds for disciplinary action by the appropriate licensing agency.
Who submits reports	All licensed medical care facilities.
Number of reports	488 (1997)
Year initiated	1986
Mandatory or voluntary	Mandatory
Access to information	All reports are confidential. All peer review information and standard of care determinations are protected under the risk management statutes. Only the facts of the case

	have been subpoenaed. The name of the reporter is protected.
Use of information	Each facility must establish a written plan for risk management and patient care quality assessment on a facility-wide basis. This initial plan must be submitted to the health department at least 60 days prior to the licensure date. The plan will be reviewed and the facility will be notified in writing concerning plan approval. The facility's governing board must review and approve the risk management plan on an annual basis. All changes must be approved by the department. Following an incident, the department will review the facility's plan to ensure that it is adequate. Depending on the severity of the incident, the department will then possibly conduct an investigation.

MASSACHUSETTS

Reportable event	Injury that is life-threatening, results in death, or requires a patient to undergo significant additional diagnostic or treatment measures. Medication errors. Major biomedical device or other equipment failure resulting in serious injury or having potential for serious injury. Surgical errors involving the wrong patient, the wrong side of the body, the wrong organ, or the retention of a foreign object. Blood transfusion errors. Any maternal death within 90 days of delivery or termination of a pregnancy. Death of a patient by suicide.
Who submits reports	All licensed health care facilities.
Number of reports	10,500 (1997); 390 were from hospitals
Year initiated	1986
Mandatory or voluntary	Mandatory

Access to information   Copies of reports submitted by facilities are available to the public after official action has been taken by the health department. The identity of the patient is removed. Reports relating to abuse, neglect, or misappropriation are confidential and are not released.

Use of information   All reports are entered into a Massachusetts Health Department database and are reviewed. This database is used to retain information on the individual case and look for general patterns across cases. Depending on the incident, the department can decide to contact the facility for more information or conduct a site visit. Deficiencies are cited if the facility is found to have not reported all relevant information.

MISSISSIPPI

Reportable event   Suicide or attempted suicide, wrongful death, unexplained injuries, abuse, and interruptions of service at the facility.

Who submits reports   All licensed health care facilities.

Number of reports   Not provided

Year initiated   1993

Mandatory or voluntary   Mandatory

Access to information   Actual reports are not accessible to the public; however statements of deficiencies and plans of correction are available by request. The health department does spend a great deal of time in litigation with malpractice attorneys who are attempting to subpoena its records.

Use of information   Attempts are made to identify trends in the data received, and the department's findings are discussed with the facility.

NEW JERSEY

Reportable event	Any incident that endangers the health and safety of a patient or employee and any death or injury associated with anesthetics.
Who submits reports	All state licensed health certificates.
Number of reports	Not provided
Year initiated	1986
Mandatory or voluntary	Mandatory
Access to information	Information is disclosed only in the event that the facility receives a citation from the state. Penalty letters revealing the name of the facility and describing the incident that led to the citation are posted on the Internet. Patient and personnel information is kept confidential.
Use of information	If deemed necessary, a state inspection team is sent to investigate the facility. The team's findings are shared with the facility, which must comply with the report's recommendations or be cited with deficiencies. Then the facility must submit a plan of correction for each deficiency. The health department can impose fines, curtail admissions, appoint a temporary manager, issue a provisional license, suspend a facility's license, or close the facility.

NEW YORK

Reportable event	An unintended adverse and undesirable development in an individual patient's condition occurring in a hospital. A list of 47 occurrences is included on a specification of reportable events.
Who submits reports	Hospitals
Number of reports	15,000–20,000 reports each year
Year initiated	1986
Mandatory or voluntary	Mandatory

Access to information	Narrative reports on incidents and the investigations conducted are protected by law, but the state can release aggregate data by hospital, including the number of reports submitted. State actions against a facility are posted on the Internet (whether the source was the reporting system, patient complaint, or other).
Use of information	The state may investigate specific incidents. If the hospital has taken action acceptable to the department, the case is closed. If the violation persists, the state may issue deficiencies or fines. The state also intends to develop regional error rates for benchmarking and dissemination to regional councils that are being formed.

OHIO

Reportable event	Death or injury resulting from equipment malfunction or treatment of the wrong subject or wrong modality.
Who submits reports	Free-standing therapy, imaging, and chemotherapy centers
Number of reports	Not provided
Year initiated	1997
Mandatory or voluntary	Mandatory
Access to information	Governed under Ohio's public record law. This law prohibits the collection of patient-specific information. The state will only be releasing aggregate data on the incidents reported. Facilities will have access only to their own information. The state plans to compile an annual report on incidents that will be available to the public.
Use of information	A database is being developed to track the number of reports received and provide an indicator of which facilities should be inves-

tigated. The goal is to identify noticeable trends in types of errors. The director of health monitors compliance and can inspect any health care provider. Health care providers may be required to regularly issue reports and undergo independent audits.

PENNSYLVANIA

Reportable event

An event that seriously compromises quality assurance or patient safety, including: deaths due to injuries, suicide, or unusual circumstances; deaths due to medication error; deaths due to malnutrition, dehydration, or sepsis; elopements; patient abuse; rape; surgery on the wrong patient or modality; hemolytic transfusion reaction; infant abduction or discharge to wrong family; fire or structural damage; unlicensed practice of a regulated profession.

Who submits reports

Hospitals, nursing homes, home health agencies, ambulatory surgical facilities, intermediate care facilities for persons with developmental disabilities.

Number of reports   Not provided

Year initiated   1990

Mandatory or voluntary Mandatory

Access to information

All collected information is confidential. Reports are often shared only with another state agency. They are not considered public material and were not intended to provide information to the public. The department usually requests that courts overrule subpoenas, and in the majority of cases its request is granted.

Use of information

On some occasions, the department will request more information from a facility and conduct investigations. This is usually done when there is a recurrence of incidents or drug misappropriation. Very few cases have resulted in a fine to a facility following an adverse event.

RHODE ISLAND

Reportable event Any incident causing or involving the following: brain injury; mental impairment; paraplegia; quadriplegia; paralysis; loss of use of limb or organ; birth injury; impairment of sight or hearing; surgery on the wrong patient; subjecting a patient to any procedure that was not ordered or intended by the physician.

Who submits reports Hospitals

Number of reports 134 (1998) from 15 facilities

Year initiated 1994

Mandatory or voluntary Mandatory

Access to information The names of personnel and patients are not disclosed in submitted reports. All reports are confidential and are protected by law. The hospital involved is contacted whenever the health department receives a subpoena from an attorney. The hospital may initiate proceedings to quash the subpoena. However, if the state takes action against the facility—for example, following a site investigation—then this information may be disclosed to the public.

Use of information Reports are reviewed by department staff and filed. If deemed warranted, an investigation of the incident will be conducted. After submitting a report the hospital must conduct a peer review process to determine whether the incident falls within the normal range of outcomes, given the patient's condition. If the hospital's findings conclude that the incident was outside the normal range, the hospital must provide the health department with the following information: an explanation of the circumstances surrounding the incident; an updated assessment of the effect of the incident on the patient; a summary of current patient status including follow-up care provided and post-incident diagnosis; and a summary of all actions taken to correct the problems identified to prevent recurrence and/or improve overall patient care. Incidents that are determined to have fallen within a normal range of outcomes by the hospital are reviewed by the health department. In the event that the health department disagrees with the hospital's findings, a separate investigation is conducted and peer review documents are examined.

SOUTH DAKOTA

Reportable event	Unnatural deaths; missing patients or residents; incidents of abuse, neglect, or misappropriation.
Who submits reports	All licensed health care facilities.
Number of reports	The health department has not kept track of the exact number of reports received. The majority are submitted by nursing homes.
Year initiated	1994
Mandatory or voluntary	Mandatory
Access to information	Reports are completely confidential, unless a deficient practice is identified at the facility. A summary of the cited deficiency is releasable information. As required by state law, a judicial court order must be issued before the health department will release any other information.

Use of information   Each incident report is analyzed to assess
whether the facility did everything possible
to avert the incident. If it did not, the facility will be cited and then they must develop
a plan of correction.

SOURCE: Information for this table was collected from each state health department by
telephone between February 24 and May 5, 1999. Each respondent was given the opportunity to review the draft and correct any errors.

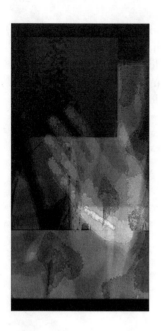

E
Safety Activities in Health Care Organizations

Numerous programs intended to promote patient safety can be found in hospitals, nursing homes, and other health care organizations. Hospitals, home health agencies, nursing homes, clinical laboratories, ambulatory surgery centers, and other health care facilities are licensed by state departments of health, which establish the terms under which they may operate.

One way in which federal and state quality oversight requirements have historically been met is through reliance on private-sector accrediting bodies, termed *deemed status*. In most circumstances, deemed status arrangements allow a facility to meet government standards either through accreditation or directly through the government agency or through accreditation by the Joint Commission on Accreditation of Healthcare Organizations (JCAHO) or the American Osteopathic Association.

A brief review of widely implemented safety programs in health care facilities, then, is grounded in the state licensing or, more likely, the voluntary accreditation standards of accrediting bodies such as the JCAHO. The JCAHO's standards for hospital accreditation,[1] for example, include several facility-wide safety systems intended to ensure patients' physical safety and protection from environmental hazards and risks, accidents, and injuries including, for example, life safety; infectious disease surveillance, prevention,

266

and control; and the handling and use of blood and blood products. Other traditional approaches to learning about error and how it might be prevented include morbidity and mortality conferences and autopsy.

LIFE SAFETY

Life safety refers to a set of standards for the construction and operation of buildings and the protection of patients from fire and smoke. These standards are based on the Life Safety Code, promulgated by the National Fire Prevention Association. Life safety standards that require fire alarm and detection systems are monitored and serviced routinely, that fire and smoke containment systems are in place, and that systems for transmitting alarms to the local fire department are functional. Facilities typically participate in fire and other disaster drills that help them identify weaknesses in their systems. By analogy, many other kinds of delivery-related simulations can probably help groups with differing disciplinary backgrounds learn to work cooperatively and effectively in, for example, the intensive care unit, emergency department, or operating room. The recent development of highly sophisticated operating room simulators has demonstrated their value both in teaching and for practitioners to practice recovering from crises.

INFECTIOUS DISEASE SURVEILLANCE, PREVENTION, AND CONTROL

Today, infection control covers a broad range of processes throughout the hospital. It requires epidemiological expertise and includes attention to medical devices (e.g., intravascular and alimentation devices, ventilators, equipment used for examination); the physical environment (e.g., air ducts, surfaces); surgical wound management; and carriage by employees and other health professionals.

Such infection control processes are managed by individuals who are assigned the responsibility of surveillance, reporting, and investigating outbreaks of nosocomial infections (infections acquired while in health care that are unrelated to the original condition), and putting in place and monitoring the results of processes to prevent or reduce the risk of infectious transmission. In the best systems, data from many sources within the hospital—infection control committee surveillance, length-of-stay outlier reports, operating room logs, bacteriology and pathology reports, morbidity and mortality (M&M) conferences and so forth—can be brought to bear to identify trends and sources of infectious disease.

Despite major efforts to decrease transmission, infection control remains a challenge to health care facilities. Indeed, in some ways it is more difficult now than in the past. Like other advances in patient care, the advent of antibiotics has dramatically improved patient care, but the emergence of antibiotic resistance means that new efforts of surveillance and prevention must be implemented in order to make progress against infection, and continuing efforts are needed to maintain earlier achievements.

According to the Centers for Disease Control (CDC), nosocomial infections affect approximately 2 million patients annually in acute care facilities in the United States at an estimated direct patient care cost of approximately $3.5 billion per year (NCID/CDC&P). In long-term care facilities including nursing homes, CDC estimates that more than 1.5 million cases of nosocomial infection occur each year, an average of one infection per patient per year.[2] Epidemiological studies have estimated that one-third of nosocomial infections can be prevented by well-organized infection control programs, yet only six to nine percent are actually prevented.

Recognition of the danger of transmission of infection in the health care setting is credited to the insight of a Viennese obstetrician Ignaz Phillip Semmelweis in 1847. Semmelweis correctly identified the cause of an epidemic of childbed fever (puerperal sepsis) among maternity patients as originating from physicians who had previously done autopsies and then transferred bacteria (later found to be *Streptococcus pyogenes*) on their hands when they examined their patients. After Semmelweis introduced the practice of hand washing with a solution of chloride of lime (an antiseptic) before examination, maternal mortality decreased from 18 percent to 2.4 percent in the first month.[3,4] According to CDC, even today, "handwashing is the single most important means of preventing the spread of infection." Yet, repeated studies indicate that after more than 150 years of experience, lack of or improper handwashing still contributes significantly to disease transmission in health care settings[5–11] Exhortations to personnel have not been effective, and some organizations have begun to look at system barriers to handwashing (e.g., the time required as well as the chapping and irritation caused by frequent handwashing) and ways to eliminate these problems by designing better hand hygiene processes.

MORBIDITY AND MORTALITY CONFERENCES

Morbidity and mortality (M&M) conferences began early in the twentieth century (1917) as a standardized case report system to investigate the reasons and responsibility for adverse outcomes of care. Mandated in 1983 by the Accreditation Council for Graduate Medical Education, M&M is a weekly conference at which, under the moderation of a faculty member, medical and surgical residents and attendings present cases of all complications and deaths. The value of the M&M conference is highly dependent on how the department chair uses it, but a recent national survey on attitudes and opinions of the value of M&M conferences found that 43 percent of residents and 47 percent of surgical faculty believed that the conference was an important and powerful educational tool.[12] Lower rankings were given to its value in reducing error and improving care.

M&M conferences are case-by-case reviews, with an emphasis on learning what might have been done differently in a given case rather than punishment, but they stress the value of knowledge, skill, and alertness to anticipate problems.[13] They tend not to address systemic issues. Their value in improving the quality of care could be substantially increased if ongoing data are kept to identify repeated complications and time trends and if information from the M&M conferences is integrated with information from other available sources within the hospital.

AUTOPSY

Unexpected findings at autopsy are an excellent way to refine clinical judgment and identify misdiagnosis. Lundberg cites a 40 percent discrepancy between antemortem and postmortem diagnoses.[14] Nevertheless, autopsy rates have declined greatly in recent years from 50 percent in the 1940s to only 14 percent in 1985.[15,16] Autopsy rates in nonteaching hospitals are now less than 9 percent.

When autopsies are completed, their value in improving care depends on reports reaching clinicians in a timely manner. Yet, many hospitals report long delays (several weeks or more) before clinicians receive autopsy reports. In general, rapid improvement requires shortening the cycle time between investigation and feedback to caregivers and managers, and timeliness in autopsy reporting is representative of all data gathering activities intended for quality improvement and reduction of errors.

RISK MANAGEMENT PROGRAMS

Originating with the increase in liability risk in the mid-1970s, hospital risk management programs have long been associated with the reduction of institutional liability and financial loss control.[17,18] Controlling loss has focused historically on preserving the institution's financial (and human) resources. Risk management includes identification of risk and education of staff, identifying and containing risk after an event, education of staff and patients, and risk transfer. Educational efforts tend to focus on such topics as review of state statutes on informed consent, presentations by the hospital's defense counsel, and programs on medical and legal topics for physicians.

Although effort has been made to move toward "primary" risk management that would focus on preventing adverse events from occurring, risk management is still focused largely on loss control. Although incident reporting systems are intended to include major events such as surgical mishaps, incidents have traditionally been greatly underreported and the reports that are filed have involved largely slips, falls, and medication errors that may have little consequence.[19,20] The American College of Surgeons estimated in 1985 that only 5–30 percent of major mishaps are reported on traditional incident forms.[21] Cullen et al. (1995) found that of 54 adverse drug events identified in their study, only six percent had a corresponding incident report submitted to the hospital's quality assurance program or the pharmacy hotline.

Although risk management committees include a member of the medical staff, risk management has not been embraced at the organizational leadership level in its broadest sense of patient safety—protecting patients from any accidental injury. Risk managers interact when necessary with the administrator or chief executive officer, medical director or chief of staff, nursing director, medical records director, and chief financial officer, but the function of improved patient safety is not, typically, represented through risk managers on the governing board's executive committee or at corporate headquarters.

REFERENCES

1. Joint Commission on Accreditation of Healthcare Organizations. *1998 Hospital Accreditation Standards*. Oakbrook, IL: Joint Commission, 1998.

2. From "Hospital Infections Program." www.cdc.gov/ncidod/publications/brochures/hip.htm 4/29/99. "Hospital Infections Program."

3. "Ignaz Philipp Semmelweis." www.knight.org/advent/cathen/1312a.htm (Catholic Encyclopedia) 4/29/99.

4. From "Etiology of Childbed Fever." www.obgyn.net/women/med-chest/med41105.htm 4/29/99.

5. Pittet, D.; Mourouga, P.; Perneger, T.V., et al. Compliance with Handwashing in a Teaching Hospital. *Annals of Internal Medicine.* 130:126–155, 1999.

6. Steere, A.C., and Mallison, G.F. Handwashing Practices for the Prevention of Nosocomial Infections. *Annals of Internal Medicine.* 83:683–690, 1975.

7. Sproat, L.J., and Inglis, T.J. A Multicentre Survey of Hand Hygiene Practices in Intensive Care Units. *Journal of Hospital Infections.* 26:137–148, 1994.

8. Albert, R.K., and Condie, F. Hand-washing Patterns in Medical Intensive-Care Units *New England Journal of Medicine.* 24:1465–1466, 1981.

9. Larson, E. Compliance with Isolation Technique. *American Journal of Infection Control.* 11:221–225, 1983.

10. Meengs, M.R.; Giles, B.K.; Chisholm, C.D., et al. Hand Washing Frequency in an Emergency Department. *Journal of Emergency Nursing.* 20:183–188, 1994.

11. Thompson, B.L.; Dwyer, D.M.; Ussery, X.T., et al. Handwashing and Glove Use in a Long-Term-Care Facility. *Infection Control and Hospital Epidemiology.* 18:97–103, 1997

12. Harbison, S.P., and Regehr, G. Faculty and Resident Opinions Regarding the Role of Morbidity and Mortality Conference. *American Journal of Surgery.* 177:136–139, 1999.

13. Gawande, A. When Doctors Make Mistakes. *The New Yorker.* 74(41):40–52, 1999.

14. Lundberg, G.D. Low-Tech Autopsies in the Era of High-Tech Medicine. *JAMA.* 280:1273–1274, 1998.

15. Geller, S.A. Autopsy. *Scientific American.* 248(3):124–129, 132, 135–136, 1983.

16. Leads from the MMWR. Autopsy Frequency—United States, 1980–1985. *JAMA.* 259:2357–2362, 1988.

17. Troyer, G.T., and Salman, S.L. *Handbook of Health Care Risk Management.* Rockville, MD: Aspen, 1986.

18. Monagle, J.F. *Risk Management: A Guide for Health Care Professionals.* Rockville, MD: Aspen, 1985.

19. Institute of Medicine. *Medicare: A Strategy for Quality Assurance,* Volume II. Washington, D.C.: National Academy Press, 1990.

20. Cullen, David J.; Bates, David W.; Small, Stephen D., et al. The Incident Reporting System Does Not Detect Adverse Drug Events: A Problem in Quality Assurance. *Joint Commission Journal on Quality Improvement.* 21:541–548, 1995.

21. Leape, Lucian, L.; Woods, David D.; Hatlie, Martin, J., et al. Promoting Patient Safety and Preventing Medical Error. *JAMA.* 280:1444–1447, 1998.

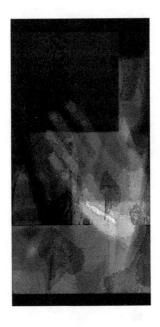

Index

273